TEACHING AND LEARNING IN NURSING

Edited by **Majda Pajnkihar, Dominika Vrbnjak** and **Gregor Štiglic**

Teaching and Learning in Nursing
http://dx.doi.org/10.5772/65314
Edited by Majda Pajnkihar, Dominika Vrbnjak and Gregor Štiglic

Contributors

Dominika Vrbnjak, Majda Pajnkihar, Klavdija Čuček Trifkovič, Barbara Donik, Sabina Fijan, Vida Gönc, Lorber Mateja, Natalya Kamynina, Irina Ostrovskaya, Kegl Barbara, Maja Strauss, Jadranka Stričević, Jasmina Nerat, Zvonka Fekonja, Milena Pišlar, Margaret Denny, Nino Fijačko, Brian Sharvin, Marget Denny, Gregor Stiglic, Nataša Mlinar Reljić, Suzanne Denieffe, Ian McGonagle, Christine Jackson, József Betlehem

Published by InTech
Janeza Trdine 9, 51000 Rijeka, Croatia

Publishing Process Manager Danijela Duric
Technical Editor SPi Global
Cover InTech Design team

First published May, 2017
Printed in Croatia
Legal deposit, Croatia: National and University Library in Zagreb

Additional hard copies can be obtained from orders@intechopen.com

Teaching and Learning in Nursing, Edited by Majda Pajnkihar, Dominika Vrbnjak and Gregor Štiglic
p. cm.
Print ISBN 978-953-51-3153-3
Online ISBN 978-953-51-3154-0

For EU product safety concerns:
IN TECH d.o.o., Prolaz Marije Krucifikse Kozulić 3, 51000 Rijeka, Croatia,
info@intechopen.com or visit our website at intechopen.com.

Meet the editors

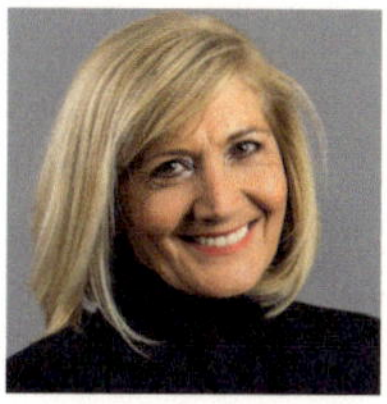

Majda Pajnkihar is a Dean, Associate Professor and Head of the Institute of Nursing Care at the University of Maribor, Faculty of Health Sciences (UM FHS). She obtained her PhD from University of Manchester in 2003 and became the first nurse with a PhD in Slovenia. She worked on numerous national and international projects in nursing and health care. She is a visiting professor at University of Osijek, Josipa Jurja Strossmayera, Medical Faculty, Department of Nursing, Osijek and was a visiting professor at University of Ulster, Belfast. Professor Pajnkihar is currently a Chair and was one of the founding members of the international UDINE-C group, connecting different nursing schools across Europe, USA and Russia. She is also an Honorary Professor at I.M. Sechenov First Moscow State Medical University and a member of Sigma Theta Tau International, Honor Society of Nursing. She received several prestigious awards for her work at the UM and a Golden badge of Nurses and Midwives Association of Slovenia.

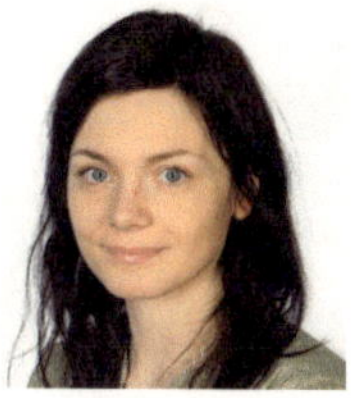

Dominika Vrbnjak is a teaching assistant at the University of Maribor, Faculty of Health Sciences. She obtained a Master degree in Nursing from University of Maribor, Faculty of Health Sciences. Currently, she is a doctoral student of Biomedical Technology at Faculty of Medicine in Maribor. During her postgraduate study, she was also a visiting PhD student of Waterford Institute of Technology in Ireland. She participates in scientific and research projects and disseminates her work in scientific papers and professional peer reviewed journals. Her research work was published in the International Journal of Nursing Studies, Journal of Nursing Management and Scandinavian Journal of Caring Sciences among others. During her undergraduate study, she received a Rector's award at the University of Maribor for the best undergraduate student in a generation. She previously worked for four years as a registered nurse at General Hospital Ptuj, where she developed communication and organizational skills while leading and coordinating the nursing care.

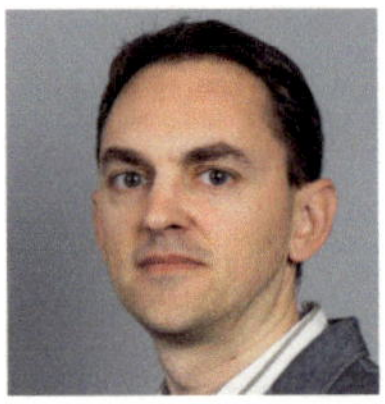

Gregor Stiglic is a Vice Dean for Research, Associate Professor and Head of Research Institute at the University of Maribor, Faculty of Health Sciences (UM FHS). He worked as a Visiting Researcher at Data Analysis and Biomedical Analytics (DABI) Center at Temple University and as a Visiting Assistant Professor at Shah Lab, Stanford School of Medicine, Stanford University. His research interests encompass application of data analytics and knowledge discovery techniques in healthcare. His work was published in multiple conference publications, peer reviewed journals and books. Dr Stiglic gave talks on his research work at renowned research institutions such as IBM T.J. Watson Research Center, Stanford University, University of Manchester, University of Edinburgh and University of Tokyo. He served as an organizer at many workshops and conferences in the field of health data science.

Contents

Preface

This book is based on the premise that there is a requirement to continually bridge the gap between nursing education and the practice of nursing. It is written by experts in the field of nursing education, practice and research. It provides unified and detailed material on teaching and learning in the field of nursing education, which is supported by evidence based practice. The material in this book is of prime interest to both nurse-educators and health care professionals who have responsibility for student/patient teaching and who wish to meet the challenges of evidence based teaching and learning in nursing, education, research and practice. We are now living in an era of change in relation to the educational process and there is a growing interest in different teaching, learning and information technology approaches that serve to motivate students to be receptive to learning. This book offers topics that are insightful, informative and practical where teaching and learning are viewed as an integrated process. It affords an opportunity for the reader to actively engage in a pedagogical process that is fundamental to integrated learning for the nursing profession and patient care.

In contemporary nursing, there is a need for an ever-growing knowledge base that should serve as a stimulus to develop innovative research and teaching in nursing education and practice. The first chapter focuses on the attitudes of nursing students to learning nurse-patient communication skills, which are often not emphasized enough in nursing education programmes and curricula. Chapter 2 provides an overview of problem based learning as an educational approach that enables students to develop essential critical thinking skills necessary for safe and effective nursing care. In Chapter 3, the authors present an approach to the development of Objective Structured Clinical Examination (OSCE), which have already been adapted by many international universities for assessment of healthcare competencies and as a formative teaching tool. The chapter discusses the measurement of the content validity of the OSCE and the process of adaptation of the checklists to the local environment. In tandem with the last chapter, Chapter 4, considers the objectivity and comprehensiveness of OSCE in comparing students' self-assessment with teacher assessment of clinical skills. Chapter 5 deals with the assessment of clinical nursing competencies by providing a critical review of the literature and describes a requirement to develop a holistic approach to clinical skills competency assessment.

The last three chapters report on developments in the clinical environment starting with Chapter 6 where the authors describe the impact of education, working conditions as well as interpersonal relationships on nurses' general job satisfaction. Chapter 7 presents an overview of the impact of psychological therapy education on practice. In the final chapter, the authors provide an overview of the characteristics of the nursing workforce in Hungary with recommendations as to how new roles can provide solutions for the current nursing shortages.

We hope that this book will serve as a resource and guide to health care professionals in fulfilling the broader role of health care education. We are thankful to several people who helped in the process of writing and editing this book. Therefore, we would like to thank all authors and reviewers, Margaret Denny, Christine Jackson, Ian McGonagle and Brian Sharvin for their hard work and especially to Margaret Denny who was always ready to help with advice and tireless help. The book was inspired by many participants of the international conference "Research and Education in Nursing" that was held in June 2016 in Maribor, hence, we would also like to thank all the staff of the Faculty of Health Science at the University of Maribor who kindly helped in organization of this successful event.

Associate Professor Majda Pajnkihar,
University of Maribor, Slovenia

Dominika Vrbnjak,
University of Maribor, Slovenia

Associate Professor Gregor Štiglic,
University of Maribor, Slovenia

Chapter 1

Attitudes of Nursing Students Towards Learning Communication Skills

Klavdija Čuček Trifkovič, Mateja Lorber,
Margaret Denny, Suzanne Denieffe and Vida Gönc

Additional information is available at the end of the chapter

http://dx.doi.org/10.5772/67622

Abstract

Introduction: Attitudes of nursing students towards learning nurse-patient communication skills have for long been a concern of lecturers, planners and policy-makers. The objectives of our study were to explore the attitudes of nursing students towards learning communication skills.

Methodology and methods: The study used a quantitative non-experimental survey. Nursing students' attitudes were assessed using the Communication Skills Attitudes Scale (CSAS), which is comprised two scales measuring positive and negative attitudes. The reliability coefficient for two subscales was calculated using Cronbach's α, with the positive attitude scale (PAS) found to be 0.855, and the negative attitude scale (NAS) 0.733.

Results: The mean score for PAS was 52.8, and the mean score for NAS was 32.7. There were no statistically significant differences identified when examining the positive attitude scale results and previous education ($t = 1.434$; $p = 0.155$) or mode of study ($t = 1.566$; $p = 0.120$), but we found statistically significant differences ($F = 10.950$; $p < 0.001$) according to the year of the study. Principal component analysis identified three factors, which explained 74% of the variance in the results.

Conclusion: CSAS measures may be helpful for monitoring the effect of different teaching strategies on students' attitudes about communication skills during nursing education. It is recommended that communication skills training programmes are designed and incorporated into all nursing curriculum.

Keywords: education, communication skills, attitudes, students, nursing

1. Introduction

Nursing is not simply the ability to successfully carry out a series of routine tasks. Instead, nursing is a holistic practice, including physical, psychological, social, environmental and political features of an illness and its impact on patients and their families. Effective communication has long been recognised as the cornerstone of high quality care in nursing as the work of healthcare is largely one of interactions and relationships [1, 2].

Communication is often taken for granted as it is a part of everyday life, yet communication, in particular competency in communication, is central to nursing. This chapter will first explore communication as a necessity in nursing. It will then consider teaching of communication skills in undergraduate healthcare programmes, exploring factors that influence this teaching. The research question will then be outlined and the research methodology described. The results of the study will then be presented. Finally, the results of the study will be compared to the key literature within the area of nursing students' attitudes towards learning communication skills.

2. Explaining communication

Communication is the transfer of information between or among people. It is not only based on an innate ability that varies from person to person, but also on the necessary training and experience that is acquired over the course of one's career.

Communication skills that have been identified as required for nursing include the following:

- verbal skills;
- non-verbal skills including awareness of body language to enable reading and interpretation of physical and emotional signs, for example, mirroring, interpreting and using non-verbal cues or the paralinguistic elements of speech;
- active listening skills demonstrating that the true listening is occurring with assimilation of information;
- voice management skills including pitch and intonation to establish and maintain rapport;
- cultural awareness including impact of the nurses own cultural background cultural sensitivity;
- written communication in practice includes clarity, coherence, knowledge of accepted medical terminology, abbreviations and acronyms.

Bramhall [3] highlights the common barriers to effective communication for the patient and nurse. Patient barriers include environmental factors such as noise, lack of privacy and lack of control over who is present; fear and anxiety; and other barriers such as an inability in articulate feelings. Nurse barriers include environmental items such as limited time, staff shortages and high workload; fear and anxiety related to causing the patient to be distressed by talking or responding to questions; and other barriers such as a lack of skills or strategies for coping with difficult emotions or queries.

3. Necessity for communication skills in nursing

The need for nurses to possess and make use of a wide range of communication skills has never been greater. Communication occurs continuously between the nurse and the patient, the patient's family, the nurse's co-workers and management. Nurses are increasingly working within multidisciplinary teams, furthering the need for advanced communication and interaction skills [4, 5].

The communication undertaken depends on the context and roles being played. Communication could include giving information, breaking news, asking or answering questions, reassuring, calming or motivating. The list is infinite, and each communication activity demands particular skills and strategies from the nurse. However, there is one underlying requirement for all communication, namely conveying the message that we value the patient as an individual who deserves to be treated with dignity and respect and good communication enables nurses to build therapeutic relationships with patients.

Communication in nursing can be a complicated process, and the possibility of sending or receiving incorrect messages frequently exists. In situations where there is poor communication, important information may not be conveyed. In the healthcare setting, poor communication can have disastrous consequences when ineffective. As many as 440,000 people die each year from preventable medical errors, representing the third leading cause of death in the United States on the list from the Centres for Disease Control [6]. Of these deaths, the Joint Commission estimated that 80% involved miscommunication.

Improving communication has been shown to be effective in reducing medical error rates. The study of Starmer et al. [7] undertaken by in the United States and Canada where medical error rates in nine children's hospitals decreased by 23% after a handoff programme was begun to enhance and standardise communication is considered.

Similarly, improving communication also increased recovery rates, increased the sense of safety and protection and improved the levels of patient satisfaction and treatment adherence [8]. Poor communication has been identified as a cause of delay and poor team performance in the care of critically ill patients [9, 10].

It is essential therefore that nurses know the key components of the communication process, how to improve on skills and the potential challenges to communication that exist.

3.1. Teaching communication skills

It has long been recognised that communication is a clinical skill and like all other clinical skills should be formally taught [11]. There is evidence that communication skills training can improve patient-centred communication, enhance empathy and provide reassurance and assist discussion of psychosocial needs [12]. Colliver et al. [13] proposed that "clinical competence and interpersonal and communication skills are related" (p. 273). They suggest that generic communication skills underlie the ability to carry out more advanced clinical skills effectively and that the confidence gained from practicing clinical skills then helps in the development of communication skills. This suggestion of a bidirectional relationship highlights the need for healthcare professional educators to ensure that education targets both specialised and generic facets of skill development.

Teaching communication skills can be undertaken in a range of methods. It has been identified through research studies that communication skills training programmes are effective if they are learner-centred, practice-oriented and have a duration of at least one day [14]. Role-play, feedback and small group discussions are effective training strategies. It is recommended that oral presentations, modelling and written information should be used as supportive strategies for this learning. It is also very important that students practise the skills they are taught. Chant et al. [15] provided an overview of education for nurses and other healthcare professionals and demonstrated the positive effects of simulated patients and experiential strategies, such as role-play and objective structured assessments.

Such a finding is confirmed by a study among nursing students undertaken by Zavertnik etal. [16] where communication skills were taught to nursing students using trained actors to portray standardised family members in a clinical learning laboratory setting. The teaching strategy was evaluated using a two-group post-test design. In addition to standard education, the intervention group received training on a communication framework and a 1-h practice session with the actor. Four domains of communication—introduction, gathering of information, imparting information and clarifying goals and expectations—were evaluated in the control and intervention groups. The intervention group performed better than the control group in all four tested domains related to communication skills. The difference with regard to the domain of gathering information was statistically significant ($p = 0.0257$). Such a study confirms that communication skills can improve and the teaching strategies used are important in determining outcomes.

Kruijver et al. [17] examined studies on communication training programmes for nurses ($n = 14$). Overall, they found limited impacts on nurses' skills, nurses' behaviours or patient outcomes. They reported that most studies had weak designs and called for experimental designs in future studies. Doyle et al. [18] in 2011 asserted that most existing studies evaluated the communication skills training for medical doctors and that more studies are needed and evaluated the effectiveness of communications training for nurses and other types of clinicians.

4. Factors impacting on learning communications skills

However, even with full consideration of teaching and assessment strategies, students may not recognise the teaching and learning of communication skills as an important part of academic education and practice. They may not perceive a need to improve their own skills in this area; instead, they may choose to focus on practical technical skills and fail to realise the true value of learning communication skills.

The attitude of the student is pivotal, and nurse educators need to know to be aware of the possible impacts of the students' attitude towards learning communication skills on the learning which occurs. Attitudes involve the creation of evaluations to which good or bad qualities of a topic/organisation or person are attached. Ajzen [19] as one of the leading attitude scientists states that an "attitude represents a summary evaluation of a psychological object captured in such attribute dimensions as good-bad, harmful-beneficial, pleasant-unpleasant, and likable-dislikeable" (p. 27). Therefore, attitudes facilitate the adaption of an individual to an environment and drive behaviour [20]. The assessment of attitudes towards patient-oriented care has its legitimation, as they refer to beliefs that are relatively stable over time [21].

Research has been under taken previously on healthcare professionals' attitudes towards learning communication skills. It seems initially that this research focused on medical student education but has moved to consideration of attitudes in many healthcare professional disciplines.

Several studies have examined attitudinal scores before and after a communication skills training [22–26]. Research using the CSAS shows different patterns of attitude development during medical education, showing decreased [27–29] to increased scores [30]. Anvik and colleagues [31] found stable cognitive attitudes in contrast to decreasing affective attitudes. Furthermore, attitudes towards communication skills appear to be less positive in students with higher levels of state anxiety [32].

Finding from Lumma-Sellenthin [33] and Molinuevo et al. [34] reproduced the gender effect known from earlier research [29, 35], wherein it was identified that female students were more positive towards communication skills training than their male peers. This was often explained by female students' stronger openness towards information-giving, partnership-building and interest in psychosocial topics.

It seems that students' positive attitudes towards learning communication skills are related to a caring patient orientation and to a good self-regulation of learning strategies [33]. However, a caring patient orientation did not depend on metacognitive abilities. Instead, it seems that the caring patient orientation was explained by a positive attitude towards communication skills learning, female gender, higher age and parents' work outside the health sector [33].

The literature has highlighted the importance of communication skills for nursing students; therefore, the aim of this cross-sectional study was to explore the attitudes of nursing students towards learning communication skills. The objective of the study was to explore both the negative and positive attitudes of nursing students towards learning communication skills.

4.1. Methodology and methods

A descriptive cross-sectional survey design was used to ascertain the attitudes of nursing students towards learning communication skills in the identified sample. The demographic variables under assessment were as follows:

- Demographic variables;
- Positive and negative attitudes towards communication skills.

The research was carried out among nursing care students of the University of Maribor, Faculty of Health Sciences in September 2016. Questionnaires (n = 342) were distributed to all nursing students. There was a 42% response rate with 143 questionnaires returned. The sample included first years (n = 75, 53%), second years (n = 18, 13%) and third years (n = 49, 34%). Of the total sample, 128 (90%) were female and 14 (10%) were male. The majority (n = 126, 89%) were full-time students, and only 16 (11%) were part-time students. Regarding previous education, 106 (75%) had finished secondary nursing school before they start study in the university with 36 (25%) having attended other secondary schools.

4.2. Ethical approval

The study procedure was approved by the Ethics Committees of the School of Health Sciences, University of Maribor. Questionnaires were not coded with an identifier; therefore, anonymity and confidentiality were assured, and this information was included in the research consent form.

4.3. Data collection tool

Nursing students' attitudes towards learning communication skills were assessed by the Nottingham Communication Skills Attitudes Scale (CSAS) questionnaire. The questionnaire contains the Interpersonal Communication Competence Scale [36] and the Communication Skills Attitude Scale (CSAS) [37]. This validated tool uses a five-point Likert scale (ranging from 1—strongly disagree to 5—strongly agree) of 13 positively (PAS) and 13 negatively (NAS) worded statements. The survey instrument uses both positive and negative statements that are intermingled throughout the questionnaire. Morris et al. [38] posits that students' scores range from 13 to 65 for PAS and 13 to 65 for NAS. The scale was developed and tested in terms of validity and reliability by Korkut [39]. In the present study, the instrument was piloted and the reliability coefficient for two subscales of CSAS was calculated using Cronbach's α. Cronbach's α for positive attitude scale (PAS) was found to be $\alpha = 0.855$, and for negative attitude scale (NAS), it was found to be $\alpha = 0.733$.

4.4. Procedure

Prior to the administration of the questionnaire, participants signed a consent form and were given the research information sheet. The online self-administered questionnaire CSAS was completed anonymously with first-, second- and third-year nursing students (n = 342) at the commencement of the first semester, September 2016. A total of 143 students participated in this study, and the response rate was 42%. Data from the completed questionnaires were analysed.

4.5. Data analysis

All scores were imported into an industry-standard software package—Statistical Package for the Social Sciences (SPSS—version 24) and statistically analysed. Descriptive statistics and inferential statistics were used to analyse the data. Demographic variables were compared using chi-squared tests. Cronbach's α was used to test the reliability coefficient for two subscales of CSAS. Statistical significance was tested using a 5% margin of error. One-way analysis of variation (ANOVA) was used to discover the differences between selected groups. A p-value of <0.05 was statistically significant.

5. Results

The mean score for PAS was 52.8 (SD = 6,7) out of 65, ranging from 30 to 65, and the mean score for NAS was 32.7 out of 65, ranging from 21 to 65.

Using independent sample t-tests, it can be seen in **Table 1** that there were no significant differences identified between males and females in either the PAS or the NAS; however, it seemed that the female students had more positive (mean score 53.0) and less negative (mean score 32.4) attitudes towards learning communication skills compared to the male students (PAS mean score 51.0; NAS mean score 35.5).

Likewise, it was identified that while there were no statistically significant differences between full- and part-time students (**Table 2**), the part-time students had more positive and also more negative attitudes towards learning communication skills compared to the group of full-time students.

It was also identified that there are no statistically significant differences between students who finished nursing or other secondary schools (**Table 3**). The group of students from other secondary schools had more positive and less negative attitudes towards learning communication skills compared to the group of students finished nursing secondary school.

Subscales	**Male**		**Female**		**t**	**p**
	Mean	**SD**	**Mean**	**SD**		
PAS	51.0	5.9	53.0	6.2	1.125	0.279
NAS	35.5	7.1	32.4	6.8	1.700	0.091

Table 1. Comparison of attitudes towards learning communication skills between male and female students.

Subscales	Full time		Part time		t	p
	Mean	SD	Mean	SD		
PAS	52.5	7.4	55.5	7.4	1.566	0.120
NAS	32.4	5.8	35.0	9.4	1.540	0.126

Table 2. Comparison of attitudes towards learning communication skills between full-time and part-time students.

Subscales	Nursing school		Other school		t	p
	Mean	SD	Mean	SD		
PAS	52.5	7.4	54.0	4.2	1.434	0.155
NAS	33.0	6.7	32.0	4.9	0.799	0.426

Table 3. Comparison of attitudes towards learning communication skills according to finished nursing and other secondary school.

There was a statistically significant difference found between the students from different programme years on the PAS (**Table 4**). Second- and third-year students had more positive and less negative attitudes towards learning communication skills compared to the first-year students.

The CSAS tool is made up of 26 questions. For the evaluation and examination of the screen chart, three factors (and all including statements) were taken into the consideration. The value of Kaiser-Meyer-Olkin test statistics was 0.860, and Bartlett's test of sphericity was significant ($p < 0.001$), both confirming the appropriateness of factor analysis.

Three factors (**Table 5**) extracted from the principal component analysis explained 74% of communication skills attitudes identified. The first, second and third factors explained 55,13 and 6%, respectively, of the entire variance. The first factor was the importance of communication skills for nursing and quality of patient care and included 12 ranked items. The second factor was the importance of learning of communication skills and included 10 ranked items. The final factor was the problem of non-acceptance of the value of learning communication skills and included 4 ranked items.

Subscales	First year		Second year		Third year		F	p
	Mean	SD	Mean	SD	Mean	SD		
PAS	50.4	6.9	56.3	5.5	55.2	5.3	10.950	<0.001
NAS	33.0	5.5	32.5	7.6	32.4	6.9	0.165	0.848

Table 4. Comparison of attitudes towards learning communication skills between students according to the study year.

http://dx.doi.org/10.5772/67622

Communication skills	IFN	LCS	PCS
Learning communication skills has helped me or will help me facilitate team-working skills	0.858	–	–
Learning communication skills has improved my ability to communicate with patients	0.757	–	–
Developing my communication skills is just as important as developing my knowledge of nursing	0.736	–	–
Learning communication skills has helped or will help me recognise patients' rights regarding confidentiality and informed consent	0.696	–	–
Learning communication skills will help me respect patients	0.671	–	–
Learning communication skills has helped me or will help me to respect my colleagues	0.662	–	–
Learning communication skills is important because my ability to communicate is a lifelong skill	0.655	–	–
When applying for nursing, I thought it was a really good idea to learn communication skills	0.641	–	–
I find it difficult to trust information about communication skills given to me by non-clinical lecturers	0.636	–	–
In order to be a good nurse, I must have good communication skills	0.538	–	–
Learning communication skills is applicable to learning nursing	0.517	–	–
Nobody is going to fail their nursing programme for having poor communication skills	0.455	–	–
Learning communication skills is interesting	–	0.771	–
I think it is really useful learning communication skills in the nursing programme	–	0.757	–
I find it difficult to take communication skills learning seriously	–	0.671	–
Communication skills teaching would have a better image if it sounded more like a science subject	–	0.641	–
Learning communication skills is fun	–	0.539	–

Communication skills	IFN	LCS	PCS
I have not got time to learn communication skills	–	0.514	–
Communication skills teaching states the obvious and then complicates it	–	0.512	–
Learning communication skills is too easy	–	0.512	–
I find it hard to admit to having some problems with my communication skills	–	0.492	–
I cannot be bothered to turn up to sessions on communication skills	–	0.469	–
I cannot see the point in learning communication skills	–	–	0.762
I do not need good communication skills to be a nurse	–	–	0.591
Communication skills learning should be left to psychology students, not nursing students	–	–	0.579
My ability to pass examinations will get me through my nursing programme rather than my ability to communicate	–	–	0.512

Note: IFN = importance for nursing and quality of patients' care; LCS = learning communication skills; PCS = problems and unacceptance of learning communication skills.

Table 5. Rotated factor matrix for three factors of learning communication skills.

6. Discussion

While it is accepted that communication skills are vital for nursing practice and that these can be learned and developed through skills training, the attitude of the student towards learning these skills is a key factor. This study has examined nursing students' attitude towards communication skills. In the research, we found that positive attitude for communication skills is in line with previous research [40–43]. In the current study, it was identified that positive attitudes towards communication skills increased slightly from the first to the second year of the nursing programme and in the last year of the programme, they decreased slightly. However, it was also identified that the negative attitude towards communication skills also decreased slightly from the first to the last year of nursing programme. An increased positive attitude towards learning communication skills depending on year of programme study was also found in previous studies [41, 42, 44]; however, Al-Bizrah et al. [40] also found that in the last year of a programme, the average scores of positive attitudes for communication skills decreased when compared with previous years of a programme.

One of main findings of our results was that communication skills were recognised as a very important part of nursing practice by the students.

In line with Neupane et al. [42], it was also identified in the current study that female students had more positive and less negative attitudes towards learning communication skills compared to male students; however, these differences were not statistically significant. This could suggest that the gender differences between the students towards communication skills identified in previous studies as being statistically significantly different is becoming less pronounced as gender roles are changing in society. Alternatively, it could be a culture-specific issue. It is certainly worthy of future exploration.

Effective communication skills for nurses are important components for today's nursing education. Furthermore, effective communication skills training programmes point to the importance of students taking an active role in the learning process [45].

A few methodological limitations require mention. The findings are based on a descriptive cross-sectional design and consequently purport to report only causal processes underlying the associations between a communication skills training and positive and negative attitudes towards a communication training in curricula. Future studies could address the idea of using a seven- or nine-point Likert scale that would yield more sensitive data [38]. Moreover, the small sample size limits the researchers' ability to make causal inferences and therefore generalisation. Future studies will require a larger more representative sample of Slovenian student nurses. The non-random selection of participants meant an available sample had to be used and the sample (n = 143) that impacted on the procedures needed to show statistically significant differences between cohorts [46]. Ultimately, measurement of communication skills, using the CSAS, at only one point [46] in time may have underestimated the effect of communication skills training in the identified cohort and consequently further limits causal inferences in this very important area of research [46].

Overall, the aim of the study undertaken was to explore the attitudes of nursing students towards learning communication skills. It was identified that the mean values for positive and negative attitudes are comparable with other research studies [40–43].

Communication skills training will remain an important component of nurse education. In line with Steckler [43], it is contended that academia needs to continue to develop and implement the use of effective communication skills to nursing students to exemplify the need for these critical skills and the importance of their part in nursing education for practice.

7. Conclusions

This study can affect the increase of interest in the specific communication skills of students and develop the departmental testing of specific communication skills of nursing students. The results of the study can be used to better prepare teachers and their students for increasing effective communication and support the recommendation that greater importance be placed on communication and the provision of more opportunities for students to learn these skills.

Acknowledgements

We would like to thank the students in the first-, second- and third-year classes of 2016 for participating in this research.

Author details

Klavdija Čuček Trifkovič[1]*, Mateja Lorber[1], Margaret Denny[1,2], Suzanne Denieffe[2] and Vida Gönc[1]

*Address all correspondence to: klavdija.cucek@um.si

1 University of Maribor Faculty of Health Sciences, Maribor, Slovenia

2 Department of Nursing and Health Care, Waterford Institute of Technology, Waterford, Ireland

References

[1] Kourkouta L, Papathanasiou IV. Communication in nursing practice. Materia Sociomedica. 2014;**26**(1):65–67. doi:10.5455/msm.2014.26.65-67

[2] Berwick DM. Escape Fire: Lessons for the Future of Health Care. New York: The Commonwealth Fund; 2002. 58 p.

[3] Bramhall E. Effective communication skills in nursing. Nursing Standard. 2014;**24**(14):53–59.

[4] King S, Carbonaro M, Greidanus E, Ansell D, Foisy-Doll C, Magus S. Dynamic and routine interprofessional simulations: expanding the use of simulation to enhance interprofessional competencies and operation of attitudes. Journal of Allied Health. 2014;**43**(3):169–175.

[5] Johnson P, Wistow G, Schulz R, Hardy B. Interagency and interprofessional collaboration in community care: the interdependence of structures and values. Medical Journal of Interprofessional Care. 2003;**17**(1):69–83. doi:10.1080/1356182021000044166

[6] James JT. A new, evidence-based estimate of patient harms associated with hospital care. Journal of Patient Safety. 2013;**9**(3):122–128. doi:10.1097/PTS.0b013e3182948a69

[7] Starmer AJ, Spector ND, Srivastava R, West DC, Rosenbluth G, Allen AD et al. Changes in medical errors after implementation of a handoff program study. The New England Journal of Medicine. 2014;**371**(19):1803–1812. doi:10.1056/NEJMsa1405556

[8] Wright R. Effective communication skills for the 'Caring' nurse [Internet]. 2012. Available from: http://www.pearsonlongman.com/tertiaryplace/pdf/ros_wright_effective_comm_skills_for_the_caring_nurse_aug2012.pdf [Accessed: 2016-12-15].

[9] Peebles E, Subbe CP, Hughes P, Gemmell L. Timing and teamwork—an observational pilot study of patients referred to a rapid response team with the aim of identifying

factors amenable to re-design of a rapid response system. Resuscitation. 2012;**83**(6):782–787. doi:10.1016/j.resuscitation.2011.12.019

[10] Andersen PO, Jensen MK, Lippert A, Østergaard DP. Identifying non-technical skills and barriers for improvement of teamwork in cardiac arrest teams. Resuscitation. 2010;**81**(6):695–702. doi:10.1016/j.resuscitation.2010.01.024

[11] Duffy FD. Dialogue: the core clinical skill. Annals of Internal Medicine. 1998;**128**(2):139–141.

[12] Sheldon LK. An evidence-based communication skills training programme for oncology nurses improves patient-centred communication, enhancing empathy, reassurance and discussion of psychosocial needs. Evidence-Based Nursing. 2011;**14**(3):87–88. doi:10.1136/ebn1156

[13] Colliver JA, Swartz MH, Robbs RS, Cohen DS. Relationship between clinical competence and interpersonal and communication skills in standardized-patient assessment. Academic Medicine. 1999;**74**(3):271–274.

[14] Berkhof M, van Rijssen HJ, Schellart AJ, Anema JR, van der Beek AJ. Effective training strategies for teaching communication skills to physicians: an overview of systematic reviews. Patient Education and Counseling. 2011;**84**(2):152–162. doi:10.1016/j.pec.2010.06.010

[15] Chant S, Jenkinson T, Randle J, Russell G, Webb C. Communication skills training in healthcare: a review of the literature. Nurse Education Today. 2002;**22**(3):189–202.

[16] Zavertnik JE, Huff TA, Munro CL. Innovative approach to teaching communication skills to nursing students. The Journal of Nursing Education. 2010;**49**(2):65–71. doi:10.3928/01484834-20090918-06

[17] Kruijver IP, Kerkstra A, Francke AL, Bensing JM, van de Wiel HB. Evaluation of communication training programs in nursing care: a review of the literature. Patient Counselling and Health Education. 2000;**39**(1):129–145.

[18] Doyle D, Copeland HL, Bush D, Stein L, Thompson S. A course for nurses to handle difficult communication situations. A randomized controlled trial of impact on self-efficacy and performance. Patient Education and Counseling. 2011;**82**(1):100–109. doi:10.1016/j.pec.2010.02.013

[19] Ajzen I. Nature and operation of attitudes. Annual Review Psychology. 2001;**52**:27–58. doi:10.1146/annurev.psych.52.1.27

[20] Eagly AH, Chaiken S. The psychology of attitudes. Fort Worth: Harcourt, Brace, & Janovich; 1993. 794 p.

[21] Wahlqvist M, Gunnarsson RK, Dahlgren G, Nordgren S. Patient-centred attitudes among medical students: gender and work experience in health care make a difference. Medical Teacher. 2010;**32**(4):e191–e198. doi:10.3109/01421591003657451

[22] Rees C, Sheard C. Evaluating first-year medical students' attitudes to learning communication skills before and after a communication skills course. Medical Teacher. 2003;**25**(3):302–307. doi:10.1080/0142159031000100409

[23] Harlak H, Gemalmaz A, Gurel FS, Dereboy C, Ertekin K. Communication skills training: effects on attitudes toward communication skills and empathic tendency. Education for Health (Abingdon, England). 2008;**21**(2):62.

[24] Bombeke K, Van Roosbroeck S, De Winter B, Debaene L, Schol S, Van Hal G et al. Medical students trained in communication skills show a decline in patient-centred attitudes: an observational study comparing two cohorts during clinical clerkships. Patient Education and Counseling. 2011;**84**(3):310–318. doi:10.1016/j.pec.2011.03.007

[25] Tiuraniemi J, Läärä R, Kyrö T, Lindeman S. Medical and psychology students' self-assessed communication skills: a pilot study. Patient Education and Counseling. 2011;**83**(2):152–157. doi:10.1016/j.pec.2010.05.013

[26] Koponen J, Pyörälä E, Isotalus P. Comparing three experiential learning methods and their effect on medical students' attitudes to learning communication skills. Medical Teacher. 2012;**34**(3):e198–e207. doi:10.3109/0142159X.2012.642828

[27] Harlak H, Dereboy C, Gemalmaz A. Validation of a Turkish translation of the Communication Skills Attitude Scale with Turkish medical students. Education for Health (Abingdon, England). 2008;**21**(1):55.

[28] Fazel I, Aghamolaei T. Attitudes toward learning communication skills among medical students of a university in Iran. Acta Medica Iranica. 2011;**49**(9):625–629.

[29] Cleland J, Foster K, Moffat M. Undergraduate students' attitudes to communication skills learning differ depending on year of study and gender. Medical Teaching. 2005;**27**(3):246–251. doi:10.1080/01421590400029541

[30] Khashab SS. Attitudes of Alexandria medical students towards communication skills learning. The Journal of the Egyptian Public Health Association. 2006;**81**(5–6):355–372.

[31] Anvik T, Grimstad H, Baerheim A, Bernt Fasmer O, Gude T, Hjortdahl P et al. Medical students' cognitive and affective attitudes towards learning and using communication skills—a nationwide cross-sectional study. Medical Teaching. 2008;**30**(3):272–279. doi:10.1080/01421590701784356

[32] Loureiro EM, Severo M, Bettencourt P, Ferreira MA. Attitudes and anxiety levels of medical students towards the acquisition of competencies in communication skills. Patient Counselling and Health Education. 2011;**85**(3):e272–e277. doi:10.1016/j.pec.2011.07.005

[33] Lumma-Sellenthin A. Students' attitudes towards learning communication skills: correlating attitudes, demographic and metacognitive variables. International Journal of Medical Education. 2012;**3**:201–208. doi:10.5116/ijme.5066.cef9

[34] Molinuevo B, Aradilla-Herrero A, Nolla M, Clèries X. A comparison of medical students', residents' and tutors' attitudes towards communication skills learning. Education for Health (Abingdon, England). 2016;**29**(2):132–135. doi:10.4103/1357-6283.188755

[35] Rees C, Sheard C. The relationship between medical students' attitudes towards communication skills learning and their demographic and education-related characteristics. Medical Education. 2002;**36**(11):1017–1027.

[36] Rubin RB, Martin MM. Development of a measure of interpersonal communication competence. Communication Research Reports. 1994;**11**(1):33–44. doi:10.1080/08824099409359938

[37] Rees C, Sheard C, Davies S. The development of a scale to measure medical students' attitudes towards communication skills learning: the Communication Skills Attitude Scale (CSAS). Medical Education. 2002;**36**(2):141–147.

[38] Morris M, Donohoe G, Hennessy M. The fall and rise of medical students' attitudes to communication skills learning in Ireland: a longitudinal approach study. British Journal of Education, Society and Behavioural Science. 2013;**3**(4):467–477. doi:10.9734/BJESBS/2013/4075

[39] Korkut F. İletişim becerileri eğitimi programının liselilerin iletişim becerilerini de ğerlendirmelerine etkisi [The impact of the communication skills training program on the communication skills of high school students]. 3P Dergisi. 2012;**4**(3):191–198.

[40] Al-Bizrah NA, Tarique NM, Arain, FR. Student attitude towards communication skills training among female medical students in Taif University. Sky Journal of Medicine and Medical Sciences. 2016;**4**(2):14–19.

[41] Ihmeideh FM, Al-Omari AA, Al-Dababneh, KA. Attitudes toward communication skills among students'-Teachers' in Jordanian Public Universities. Australian Journal of Teacher Education. 2010;**35**(4). doi:10.14221/ajte.2010v35n4.1

[42] Neupane MS, Neupane HC, Adhikari S, Aryal B. Attitude towards learning communication skills in medical students of Chitwan Medical College, Chitwan, Nepal. International Journal of Pharmaceutical and Biological Archives. 2012;**3**(5):1058–1061.

[43] Steckler R. Improving communication skills among nursing students: assessing the Comfort Curriculum as an intervention [thesis]. Lexington: University of Kentucky; 2012. 64 p. Available from: http://uknowledge.uky.edu/cgi/viewcontent.cgi?article=1006&context=comm_etds

[44] Laurence B, Bertera EM, Feimster T, Hollander R, Stroman C. Adaptation of the Communication Skills Attitude Scale (CSAS) to dental students. Journal of Dental Education. 2012;**76**(12):1629–1638.

[45] Fallowfield L, Jenkins V, Farewell V, Saul J, Duffy A, Eves R. Efficacy of a cancer research UK communication skills training model for oncologists: a randomised controlled trial. The Lancet. 2002;**359**:650–656.

[46] Denny M, Wells J, Cunningham J. Assessing psychosocial work-related stress across five European countries: implications for workforce development. The Journal of Mental Health Training, Education and Practice. 2012; **6**(2), 93–103.

Chapter 2

Experience of Problem-Based Learning for Raising Quality of Nursing Study

Vida Gönc, Mateja Lorber and Jasmina Nerat

Additional information is available at the end of the chapter

http://dx.doi.org/10.5772/67427

Abstract

Introduction: Problem-based learning is a teaching method that encourages critical thinking, group interaction, and application of the theory into practice. Transition to active forms of learning, with integrating problem-solving strategies, will help to raise the quality of education. The aim of the study is to determine students' evaluation of problem-based learning in the study of nursing.

Methods: Descriptive method and quantitative research methodology were used. Nursing students from one of the faculties in Slovenia participated in the study and structured questionnaires (Cronbach $\alpha = 0.953$) were used.

Results: Average values of all items regarding to the student's evaluation of problem-based learning were very high (>4 out of 5). According to the results, there is no statistically significant difference in the assessment of problem-based learning between full-time and part-time students ($t = -0.818$, $p = 0.414$), but we found statistically significant differences ($t = 2.377$, $p = 0.018$) depending on whether students are employed in nursing or not.

Discussion and conclusion: Problem-based learning encourages nursing students' motivation, independence, and teamwork and helps to acquire knowledge and skills necessary to function in nursing.

Keywords: problem-based learning, learning, students, nursing

1. Introduction

According to the demographic changes of the population, increasing numbers of older people, the rapid changes, and innovations in the field of health care, as well as increasing numbers of people with chronic illnesses, nursing has an increasingly important role [1].

Changes in nursing require from nurses, autonomy and the ability to take relevant decisions [2], therefore, is one of the goals of nursing education to reduce the gap between theory and practice [3, 4]. For an effective transfer of theoretical knowledge into practice, changes are needed. According to Shuler [5], it is necessary to change traditional teaching into the active form of teaching. One of the active ways of learning is problem-based learning. This is an innovative educational method [6, 7] which encourages critical thinking and group interaction and represents an advantage compared to traditional ways of teaching, because it integrates problem-solving strategies [8]. Characteristics of problem-based learning are student-centered learning, learning in smaller groups and acquiring new information with self-learning [9]. Problem-based learning improves students' learning and simultaneously helps with problem-solving in everyday life [10]. With the problem-based learning approach, the activity of learning starts with a problem that describes phenomena or events needed for understanding [11]. Simultaneously, the problem-based learning approach activates students' previous knowledge [6].

For a successful problem-based learning after Munshi et al. [12], quality shaped and selected problems are key elements. Research studies [5, 13, 14] showed that information gained with problem-solving ways of learning is preserved longer. Therefore, in the opinion of authors [13, 15–17], learning based on problem-solving develops skills of communication, problem-solving, teamwork, leadership, and understanding; skills that are important for smoother transition into a clinical environment.

The purpose of the study is to determine the evaluation of problem-based learning, and the problems with which nursing students face in problem-based learning.

1.1. Methods

A quantitative research method was used. We used a structured questionnaire containing 20 statements regarding students' evaluation of ways of learning based on problems and demographic data (sex, age, type of study, and employment status in nursing). Students' views on the effectiveness of problem-based learning were assessed by using 20 items from the problem-based learning evaluation questionnaire [17], which was partially adapted and prepared in Slovenian language. Problem-based learning evaluation questionnaires were already used in studies [17–19]. Using the questionnaire, we evaluated five key dimensions of problem-based learning: construction of professional knowledge, development of problem-solving skills, development of self-directed learning, improvement of motivation, and promotion of effective group collaboration. Each of the studied dimensions contained four items and participants responded on the five-point Likert's scale ranging from (1 – strongly disagree, 2 – disagree, 3 – neutral, 4 – agree to 5 – strongly agree). The instrument's internal consistency using Cronbach's alpha was 0.80 and the test-retest reliability with a 2-week interval was 0.89 [17]. The Cronbach's alpha for our questionnaire was 0.953.

1.2. Sample description

The research was carried out among nursing students of the University of Maribor Faculty of Health Sciences. A total of 198 questionnaires were handed out, and 196 were returned which is a 98.9% response. In the research, 101 (51.5%) first-year students and 92 (47.0%) second-year students participated, three (1.5%) students did not state their year of study. Average age of participants was 21.2 years (ages between 19 and 42). 146 (74.5 %) participants were of full-time study where 76 (38.7%) were first-year students and 70 (35.8 %) were second-year students. Forty-seven (25.5 %) participants were of part-time study where twenty-five were first-year students (12.8 %) and twenty-two (11.2%) were second-year students. Three (1.5%) students did not write down their type of study. Among the part-time students only 18 students employed in nursing, but other 27 part-time students and all full-time students (146) are not employed in nursing. Two (1%) part-time students did not write if they are employed in nursing or not.

1.3. Description of research procedure

Before we started to execute the research we obtained written agreements from University of Maribor Faculty of Health Sciences leadership and University of Maribor Faculty of Health Sciences Commission for Ethical Questions from the Field of Nursing Care. Based on the agreement the research was carried out in academic year 2013–2014 and academic year 2014–2015 at course nursing care of women with gynecology and obstetrics and management of hospital infections. At selected course, we started carrying out problem-based learning in 2011.

Participants were informed with purpose and aims of the research. Participation was voluntary and anonymous. Questionnaires were handed out after completing all course obligations of selected courses. Data was processed by the statistical computer program SPSS 20.0. We used descriptive statistics and t-test to discover differences between two groups. A p-value of < 0.05 was considered significant.

2. Results

Average values of all items regarding to the student's evaluation of problem-based learning were very high (>4 out of 5). The lowest average value (4.06) was in item that problem situations encouraged students to continue to study on their own and the highest average values (4.54) were in item that the content of the course is useful for student's future work. Evaluation of problem-based learning dimensions was assessed by students with average value 4.29 (4.26–4.42). The lowest average values received dimensions "development of self-directed learning" (4.26) and "improving motivation" (4.26). The highest average value received the dimension "promotion of effective group collaboration" (4.42). **Table 1** represents results of average values of evaluation of problem-based learning.

With the t-test we want to find out if there are any statistically significant differences of evaluation of five dimension of problem-based learning regarding the type of study (full-time/part-time) and found out that none of the examined dimensions "construction of professional knowledge" ($t = 1.194$, $p = 0.234$), "development of problem-solving skills" ($t = 1.010$, $p = 0.314$), "development of self-directed learning" ($t = 0.418$, $p = 0.676$), "improvement of motivation" ($t = 1.605$, $p = 0.110$), and "promotion of effective group collaboration" ($t = 0.384$, $p = 0.701$) not show statistical significant differences (**Table 2**).

Items for evaluation of problem-based learning	1 Strongly disagree N(%)	2 Agree N(%)	3 Neutral N(%)	4 Agree N(%)	5 Strongly agree N(%)	Mean (SD)
The course made me use previous relevant knowledge and experience.	0(0)	3(2)	26(13)	85(44)	81(41)	4.25 (0.742)
The course helped me to interpret, analyze and apply key concepts precisely.	0(0)	4(2)	14(7)	103(54)	74(38)	4.27 (0.682)
The course furthered my in-depth understanding of nursing knowledge.	1(1)	0(0)	14(7)	84(43)	96(48)	4.41 (0.670)
The content of the course is useful for my future work.	1(1)	1(1)	10(5)	63(32)	119(61)	4.54 (0.668)
Construction of professional knowledge						4.363 (0.561)
The problem use in the course was challenging to discuss.	0(0)	6(3)	15(8)	77(39)	97(50)	4.36 (0.756)
The course increased my ability to solve real-world problems.	2(1)	4(2)	22(12)	82(42)	84(43)	4.25 (0.813)
The course encouraged me to consider alternatives when solving problems.	1(1)	3(2)	24(12)	78(40)	89(45)	4.29 (0.780)
The course helped me to take reasonable inferences and conclusions.	2(1)	4(2)	21(11)	72(37)	96(49)	4.31 (0.825)
Development of problem-solving skills						4.3 (0.690)
Problem situations encouraged me to continue to study on my own.	1(1)	9(4)	37(19)	78(40)	70(36)	4.06 (0.883)
The course helped me to identify gaps in my knowledge.	1(1)	3(2)	23(12)	80(41)	88(44)	4.29 (0.773)
The course helped me improve my ability to identify a variety of resources.	2(1)	5(3)	27(14)	80(41)	81(41)	4.19 (0.745)
The course helped me to think independently.	0(0)	2(1)	15(8)	62(32)	115(59)	4.50 (0.686)
Development of self-directed learning						4.26 (0.687)
The course encouraged me to take an active role in my learning.	1(1)	6(3)	19(10)	82(42)	87(44)	4.27 (0.801)
The course motivated me to learn more.	1(1)	8(4)	19(10)	82(42)	85(43)	4.24 (0.830)
The course stimulated my interest in learning.	3(2)	7(4)	23(12)	80(41)	82(42)	4.18 (0.889)
The course encouraged my participation through the discussion of problems.	2(1)	0(0)	20(10)	85(44)	89(45)	4.32 (0.741)
Improvement of motivation						4.26 (0.706)
The course stimulated group discussion.	2(1)	3(2)	13(6)	64(33)	113(58)	4.45 (0.774)
The course promoted open discussion of differing opinions.	1(2)	2(1)	18(9)	62(31)	111(57)	4.44 (0.748)

Items for evaluation of problem-based learning	1 Strongly disagree N(%)	2 Agree N(%)	3 Neutral N(%)	4 Agree N(%)	5 Strongly agree N(%)	Mean (SD)
The course increased my ability to work effectively on a team.	2(1)	7(4)	20(10)	66(34)	100(51)	4.31 (0.871)
The course encouraged me to share what I learned with the entire group.	0(0)	3(2)	15(8)	63(32)	114(58)	4.48 (0.707)
Promotion of effective group collaboration						4.42 (0.651)

Table 1. Results of evaluation of problem-based learning.

	Type of study	Min	Max	Mean	SD	*t*	*p*	df
Construction of professional knowledge	Full-time	1.5	5	4.34	0.587	1.194	0.234	189
	Part-time	3.25	5	4.45	0.464			
Development of problem-solving skills	Full-time	1.25	5	4.27	0.704	1.010	0.314	190
	Part-time	3.0	5	4.39	0.657			
Development of self-directed learning	Full-time	1.5	5	4.25	0.66	0.418	0.676	188
	Part-time	2.5	5	4.29	0.738			
Improvement of motivation	Full-time	1	5	4.2	0.717	1.605	0.110	190
	Part-time	2.25	5	4.39	0.671			
Promotion of effective group collaboration	Full-time	2.75	5	4.43	0.629	0.384	0.701	189
	Part-time	2	5	4.39	0.727			
Evaluation of problem-based learning	Full-time	1.6	5	4.3	0.574	0.818	0.414	186
	Part-time	2.85	5	4.37	0.551			

Table 2. Results of *t*-test for problem-based learning according to the type of study.

With the *t*-test we also tested statistical significant differences regarding employment or unemployment in nursing and found out there are statistically significant differences of two studied dimensions, "development of problem-solving skills" ($t = 2.197$, $p = 0.029$) and "development of self-directed learning" ($t = 4.443$, $p < 0.001$), whereas at "promotion of effective group collaboration" ($t = 1.699$, $p = 0.091$), "improvement of motivation" ($t = 1.493$, $p = 0.121$), and "construction of professional knowledge" ($t = 2.180$, $p = 0.052$), we did not find statistical significant differences among students that are employed or not employed in nursing (**Table 3**).

Regarding to the total grade of average values for all five dimensions of problem-based learning from the students' point of view, we found out statistically significant differences regarding employment status (employed or not employed) in nursing ($t = 2.377$, $p = 0.018$), whereas regarding the type of study, we did not find statistical significant differences ($t = 0.818$, $p = 0.414$) at the total grade of average value for problem-based learning. On the open-ended question, students noted next difficulties with problem-based learning: lack of knowledge and information, unequal participation in the group, and the difficulty in finding literature.

Dimension of problem-based learning	Employ in nursing	Min	Max	Mean	SD	*t*	*p*	df
Construction of professional knowledge	Yes	3.25	5	4.61	0.494	2.180	0.052	190
	No	1.5	5	4.34	0.564			
Development of problem-solving skills	Yes	3.75	5	4.64	0.439	**2.197**	**0.029**	191
	No	1.25	50	4.27	0.705			
Development of self-directed learning	Yes	4	5	4.68	0.381	**4.443**	**<0.001**	189
	No	1.5	5	4.21	0.688			
Improvement of motivation	Yes	2.5	5	4.5	0.737	1.493	0.121	191
	No	1	5	4.22	0.700			
Promotion of effective group collaboration	Yes	3.5	5	4.67	0.514	1.699	0.091	189
	No	2	5	4.39	0.662			
Evaluation of problem-based learning	Yes	3.8	5	4.62	0.394	**2.377**	**0.018**	175
	No	1.6	5	4.29	0.757			

Table 3. Results of *t*-test for problem-based learning according to employment in nursing.

3. Discussion and conclusion

The research showed that average values regarding all five dimensions of problem-based learning are high. Regarding to the average values, we determined that students recognize the meaning of problem-based-learning approach in effective learning, active cooperation, teamwork, improvement of communication skills, recognition of own learning needs, and transfer of theoretical knowledge into nursing practice, what was also stated as important dimensions of problem-based learning by Yuan et al. [20] and Tseng et al. [21].

Although average values of all dimensions are high, we can agree with Luh et al. [22] regarding to the dimension "construction of professional knowledge" where they state that acquisition of professional knowledge and professional development influences students' previous knowledge and a high degree of thinking ability. On the other hand, problem-based learning helps students to provide professional knowledge and the thinking ability. The importance of previous knowledge and experience also indicates statistically significant difference in the average values of some dimensions of evaluation of problem-based learning, assessed by the students employed in nursing. Despite the fact we have to explain the results with the caution, since in the group of employed students were involved only 18 students. Based on the results, we can conclude that part-time students, who have work experiences in nursing, are more effective at problem solving and with that connected independent learning.

The difficulties of the students, which referred to those students who do not want to cooperate, or unequally cooperate with the group, and the problems of selecting participating students were already pointed by Visschers-Pleijers et al. [23] who stated the importance of selecting a group of appropriate size. Students also identified as a problem, worse understanding of the problem, as already noted by Marentič-Požarnik [24]. We confirmed that students with work experience in nursing are more efficient at problem-solving and independent learning.

The research indicates the need for problem-based learning with the goal of encouraging independent and active learning and the opportunity for students to make suggestions in the study process. Based on evaluation of teaching methods, higher education teachers can prepare improvement plans. Skinder Savić and Kaučič [25] stated that a quality course and connection of theoretical and practical starting points are key elements for achieving competencies in nursing.

We can finish with the thought that problem-based learning stimulates in students an independent and individual study process, group work, improves work motivation, and communication skills. Problem-based learning stimulates at students the sense for a responsible acquiring of professional knowledge and development of problem-solving skills.

Author details

Vida Gönc*, Mateja Lorber and Jasmina Nerat

*Address all correspondence to: vida.goenc@um.si

Faculty of Health Sciences, University of Maribor, Maribor, Slovenia

References

[1] Thiekötter A. Changing tasks for nurses in everyday practice: what type of education and research do we need? In: Skela-Savič B, Kaučič BM, Filej B, editors. Novi trendi v sodobni zdravstveni negi – razvijanje raziskovanja, izobraževanja in multisektorskega partnerskega sodelovanja: zbornik predavanj z recenzijo. 2. mednarodna znanstvena konferenca s področja raziskovanja v zdravstveni negi in zdravstvu; 17–18 September 2009; Ljubljana. Jesenice: Visoka šola za zdravstveno nego; 2009. pp. 114–121.

[2] Billings DM, Halstead JA, editors. Teaching in nursing: a guide for faculty. 3rd ed. St. Louis: Saunders/Elsevier; 2009. 541 p.

[3] Tiwari A, Chan S, Wong E, Wong D, Chui C, Wong A, et al. The effect of problem-based learning on students' approaches to learning in the context of clinical nursing education. Nurse Education Today. 2006;**26**(5):430–438.

[4] Etheridge SA. Learning to think like a nurse: stories from new nurse graduates. Journal of Continuing Education in Nursing. 2007;**38**(1):24–30.

[5] Shuler CF. Comparisons in basic science learning outcomes between students in PBL and traditional dental curricula at the same dental school. In: Bridges S, Colman McGrath T, Whitehill L, editors. Problem-based learning in clinical education: the next generation. London: Springer; 2012. pp. 35–46.

[6] Kong LN, Qin B, Zhou YQ, Mou SY, Gao HM. The effectiveness of problem-based learning on development of nursing students' critical thinking: a systematic review and

meta-analysis. International Journal of Nursing Studies. 2014;**51**(3):458–469. DOI: 10.1016/j.ijnurstu.2013.06.009

[7] Martyn J, Terwijn R, Kek MY, Huijser H. Exploring the relationships between teaching, approaches to learning and critical thinking in a problem-based learning foundation nursing course. Nurse Education Today. 2014;**34**(5):829–835. DOI: 10.1016/j.nedt.2013.04.023

[8] Wang JJ, Lo CH, Ku YL. Problem solving strategies integrated into nursing process to promote clinical problem solving abilities of RN-BSN students. Nurse Education Today. 2004;**24**(8):589–595.

[9] DeYoung S. Teaching strategies for nurse educators. 2nd ed. New Jersey: Prentice Hall; 2009. 320 p.

[10] Niemer L, Pfendt K, Gers M. Problem-based learning in nursing education: a process for scenario development. Nurse Educator. 2010;**35**(2):69–73. DOI: 10.1097/NNE.0b013e3181ced891

[11] Wood DF. Problem based learning. British Medical Journal. 2008;**336**(7651):971. DOI: 10.1136/bmj.326.7384.328

[12] Munshi FM, El Sayed AZE, Dolmans DH. Development and utility of a questionnaire to evaluate the quality of PBL problems. South East Asian Journal of Medical Education. 2008;**2**(2):32–40.

[13] Chikotas NE. Problem-based learning and clinical practice: the nurse practitioners' perspective. Nurse Education in Practice. 2009;**9**(6):393–397. DOI: 10.1016/j.nepr.2009.01.010

[14] Cheng CY, Liou SR, Tsai HM, Chang CH. The effects of team-based learning on learning behaviors in the maternal-child nursing course. Nurse Education Today. 2014; **34**(1):25–30. DOI: 10.1016/j.nedt.2013.03.013

[15] Hung W. Enhancing systems-thinking skills with modeling. British Journal of Educational Technology. 2007;**38**(1):24–30.

[16] Postholm MB. Group work as a learning situation: a qualitative study in a university classroom. Teachers and Teaching: Theory and Practice. 2008;**14**(2):143–155.

[17] Yuan HB, Williams BA, Yin L, Liu M, Fang J, Pang D. Nursing students' views on the effectiveness of problem-based learning. Nurse Education Today. 2011;**31**(6):577–581. DOI: 10.1016/j.nedt.2010.10.009

[18] Al-Kloub MI, Salameg, TN, Froelicher ES. Nursing students' evaluation of problem based learning and the impact of culture on the learning process and outcomes: a pilot project. Nurse Education in Practice. 2014;**14**(2):142–147. DOI: 10.1016/j.nepr.2013.06.013

[19] Keshk LI, El-Azim SA, Qalawa SA. Quality of problem based learning scenarios at College of nursing in Egypt and KSA: comparative study. American Journal of Education Research. 2016;**4**(9):701–710. DOI: 10.12691/education-4-9-10

[20] Yuan H, Williams BA, Fan L. A systematic review of selected evidence on developing nursing students' critical thinking through problem-based learning. Nurse Education Today. 2004;**28**(6):657–663. DOI: 10.1016/j.nedt.2007.12.006

[21] Tseng HC, Chou FH, Wang HH, Ko HK, Jian SY, Weng WC. The effectiveness of problem-based learning and concept mapping among Taiwanese registered nursing students. Nurse Education Today. 2011;**31**(8):e41–e46. DOI: 10.1016/j.nedt.2010.11.020

[22] Luh SP, Yu MN, Lin YR, Chou MJ, Chou MC, Chen JY. A study on the personal traits and knowledge base of Taiwanese medical students following problem-based learning instructions. Annals Academy of Medicine Singapore. 2007;**36**(9):743–750.

[23] Visschers-Pleijers AJ, Dolmans DH, Wolfhagen IH, van der Vleuten CP. Development and validation of a questionnaire to identify learning-oriented group interactions in PBL. Medical Teacher. 2005;**27**(4):375–381.

[24] Marentič-Požarnik B. Problemsko zasnovan študij. In: Mihevc B, Marentič-Požarnik B, Kejžar I, editors. Za boljšo kakovost študija: pogovori o visokošolski didaktiki. Ljubljana: Center za pedagoško izobraževanje Filozofske fakultete, Slovensko društvo za visokošolsko didaktiko; 1998. pp. 123–129.

[25] Skinder Savič K, Kaučič BM. Evalvacija kabinetnih vaj pri predmetu zdravstvena nega otroka in mladostnika s strani študentov Visoke šole za zdravstveno nego Jesenice. Obzornik Zdravstvene Nege. 2010;**44**(4):231–237.

Chapter 3

Using Content Validity for the Development of Objective Structured Clinical Examination Checklists in a Slovenian Undergraduate Nursing Program

Nino Fijačko, Zvonka Fekonja, Margaret Denny, Brian Sharvin, Majda Pajnkihar and Gregor Štiglic

Additional information is available at the end of the chapter

http://dx.doi.org/10.5772/intechopen.68454

Abstract

Introduction: The objective structured clinical examination (OSCE) has been adopted by many universities for the assessment of healthcare competencies and as a formative teaching tool in both undergraduate and postgraduate nursing education programs. This pilot study evaluates the validity of OSCE checklists to be used in first-year undergraduate nurse practice education.

Methods: The study involved two interconnected methodological phases. In phase one, the degree of complexity phase, essential nursing skills were estimated by a 10-point scale. In phase two, the content validity index phase, the most complex essential nursing skills in nursing were estimated by a four-point scale for analyzing content validity for each item.

Results: Nursing educators from the University of Maribor in Slovenia systematically selected and evaluated 6 out of 72 essential nursing skills for developing OSCE checklists. Peripheral cannula insertion was estimated as a skill of "very high complexity" and was used to estimate the content validity index (CVI). For peripheral cannula insertion, it was found that the item-level content validity index for 39 items was ranging from 0.82 to 1.00, which is considered as good content validity evidence.

Discussion and conclusions: Findings from the CVI analysis are promising for developing standardized checklists for OSCE and look promising for further research using OSCE as an assessment modality.

Keywords: objective structured clinical examination, development, checklist, content validity index, nursing

1. Introduction

The objective structured clinical examination (OSCE) was originally developed for medical education in Scotland by Harden and colleagues in 1975 [1], but has now been widely accepted as a "fit-for-purpose" instrument for measuring clinical skills competency in healthcare education [2, 3]. The OSCE is defined as "an approach to the assessment of clinical competence in which the components of competence are assessed in a well-planned or structured way with attention being paid to objectivity" [4].

The OSCE has been adopted by many universities for the assessment of healthcare competencies, and it is generally accepted as a valid assessment tool and as a formative teaching approach in both undergraduate and postgraduate nursing education programs [5–8]. The benefits accrued by using the OSCE tool include the development of students' confidence [5]; the preparation of students for clinical practice [9]; the achievement of deeper and more meaningful learning [7]; the ability to provide students with feedback on their clinical skills performance; and additionally its enables students to identify their strengths and weaknesses in clinical skills [6].

The OSCE typically consists of a circuit or series of short assessment tasks, each of which is assessed by an examiner using a predetermined, objective marking scheme to make the assessment of clinical skills more objective rather than subjective [10]. In an OSCE, each student has to demonstrate specific skills and behaviors in a simulated environment. The OSCE acronym has itself evolved over the years, and there are now many variations, for example, Group Objective Structured Clinical Examination [11], Objective Structured Video Exam [12], Objective Structured Assessment of Technical Skill [13], Objective Structured Teaching Encounter [14], etc. The latter number of variations on the OSCE has evolved because of its utility and applicability as an assessment and teaching tool in nursing and interprofessional education [15].

The development of new criteria for assessing clinical skills requires critical scrutiny to ensure that the validity and reliability of each assessment are maximized [10]. Validity focuses on whether a test actually succeeds in addressing the competencies it is designed to test [16]. The assessment checklists used in the OSCE are developed according to evidence-based practice guidelines and standards of nursing care to establish content validity [17]. Evaluating content validity is a critical early step in enhancing the construct validity of an instrument, and therefore, content validation is an important topic for clinicians and researchers who require high-quality measurements [18]. The content validity index (CVI) based on expert ratings of relevance is the most widely used method among nurse researchers of quantifying content validity for multi-item scales [10].

This study describes two interconnected methodological phases that could be considered and implemented when developing and establishing the CVI of a checklist, which is designed to measure nursing student performance during clinical skills assessment using OSCE. Checklists in an OSCE provide an ideal method for assessing skills that require a series of steps that should be completed with consistency and continuity each time the skill is performed [20].

2. Methods

The checklist for the OSCE was developed in three methodological and chronological phases (**Figure 1**).

In first phase, a comprehensive search of the literature relating to OSCE in Slovenian nursing was conducted and no published research examining the use of OSCE in Slovenian nursing curriculum was found.

In second phase, the degree of complexity (DOC) phase, a 10-point scale was created and used to evaluate the DOC for each essential nursing skill as perceived by nursing educators. All essential nursing skills that were included in this study were part of a first-year curriculum in the practical nursing education at one of University in Slovenia.

The DOC has 10 levels in which 1 represents "very low complexity" and 10 represents "very high complexity." The DOC scores for each essential nursing skill were classified into three categories. A score between 1 and 4 belonged to the low complexity category; a score between 4 and 8 belonged to the medium complexity category, and a score between 8 and 10 belonged to the high-complexity category.

Phase three, the content validity index (CVI) phase, included various measurements [18]. Educators evaluated each item in nursing procedures by using a four-point Likert-type ordinal scale in which 1 = not relevant, 2 = somewhat relevant, 3 = quite relevant, 4 = highly relevant, nurse. Two metrics were calculated in the scope of CVI analysis: (1) Item Content Validity

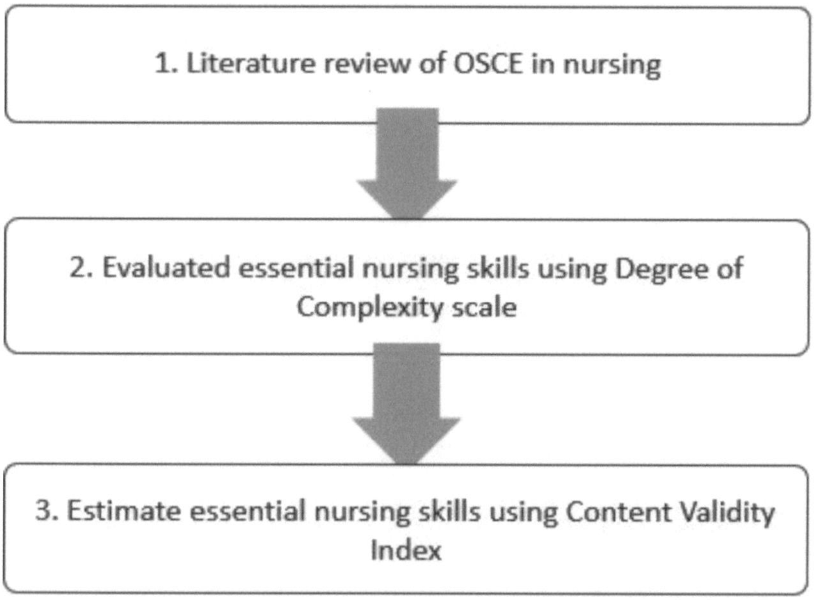

Figure 1. Methodological and chronological phases of developing checklist for the OSCE.

Index (I-CVI) and (2) Content Validity Index Average (S-CVI/Ave). The first metric (I-CVI) represents the count of all items in the essential nursing skill, which were rated with 3 or 4 divided by the total number of nursing educators. The S-CVI/Ave was calculated after summing all I-CVI numbers and dividing them by the number of items in the essential nursing skill [18].

3. Results

Nursing educators (n = 12) systematically evaluated seventy-two essential nursing skills using a 10-point DOC scale. The average DOC score for each procedure was then rearranged into one of three categories (low, medium and high). Twelve essential nursing skills with an average DOC score of 3.44 (95% confidence interval (CI): 3.07–3.82) were ranked in the low complexity category, forty-six essential nursing skills with an average DOC score of 5.84 (CI: 5.55–6.12) in the medium complexity category, and fourteen essential nursing skills with an average DOC score of 8.54 (CI: 8.36–8.71) in the high-complexity category.

Table 1 presents the essential nursing skills (n = 14) with average DOC scores from highest to lowest in the high-complexity category. Peripheral cannula insertion and female urinary

Essential nursing skills	Areas in nursing	Average degree of complexity score
Peripheral cannula insertion	Diagnostic/therapeutic essential nursing skills	9.00
Urinary catheterization: female	Elimination	9.00
Suctioning the nasopharyngeal airway	Respiratory care	8.75
Medication: injection of intravenous drugs	Medical management	8.75
Suctioning the oropharyngeal airway	Respiratory care	8.67
Tracheostomy: suctioning a patient	Respiratory care	8.67
Endotracheal suctioning of the adult intubated patient with open suction systems	Respiratory care	8.67
Venipuncture	Diagnostic/therapeutic essential nursing skills	8.50
Cleaning infected wound	Diagnostic/therapeutic essential nursing skills	8.50
Nursing care of tracheostomy	Respiratory care	8.33
Insertion of a nasogastric tube	Nutrition	8.25
Pressure Ulcer Treatment	Diagnostic/therapeutic essential nursing skills	8.18
Mouth care in unconscious patients	Personal hygiene	8.17
Rinsing infected wound	Diagnostic/therapeutic essential nursing skills	8.08

Table 1. Ranking of essential nursing skills from highest to lowest by average degree of complexity score in high-complexity category.

catheterization were estimated with the highest average DOC score (9.00 or "very high complexity"). In the DOC, phase essential nursing skills were also arranged into areas in nursing.

Nursing essential nursing skills (n = 6) with the highest average DOC score in each separate nursing areas were used for further estimate by CVI phase. Eleven nursing educators estimate I-CVI for each essential nursing skill with different number of items (range from 28 to 58). For peripheral cannula insertion, I-CVI was calculated for 39 of items and ranged from 0.82 to 1.00, which represents a good content validity. None of the items were deleted during CVI because they met agreements recommended by Polit and colleagues (**Table 2** and **Figure 2**) [19].

Item	E1	E2	E3	E4	E5	E6	E7	E8	E9	E10	E11	Number of experts	I-CVI
1	4	2	4	4	4	4	4	4	1	4	4	11	0.82
2	4	2	3	4	4	4	4	4	1	4	4	11	0.82
3	4	3	4	4	4	4	4	4	2	4	4	11	0.91
4	4	4	4	4	4	4	4	4	4	4	4	11	1.00
5	4	3	4	4	4	4	3	4	3	4	4	11	1.00
6	4	4	3	4	4	4	3	3	3	4	4	11	1.00
7	4	4	4	4	4	4	4	4	4	4	4	11	1.00
8	3	2	3	4	1	4	3	4	3	4	4	11	0.82
9	4	3	4	4	4	4	4	4	2	4	4	11	0.91
10	4	3	4	4	4	4	4	3	4	4	4	11	1.00
11	4	2	4	4	3	4	4	3	3	4	4	11	0.91
12	4	3	4	4	3	4	4	4	2	4	4	11	0.91
13	3	2	3	4	3	4	3	4	2	4	3	11	0.82
14	4	3	4	4	4	4	4	4	3	4	4	11	1.00
15	4	4	4	4	2	4	4	3	4	4	4	11	0.91
16	4	4	4	4	4	4	4	4	4	4	4	11	1.00
17	3	4	3	4	3	4	4	4	2	4	3	11	0.91
18	4	3	4	4	4	4	4	4	3	4	4	11	1.00
19	4	3	4	4	4	4	3	4	4	4	4	11	1.00
20	4	3	4	4	4	4	4	4	4	4	4	11	1.00
21	4	3	4	4	4	4	4	4	4	4	4	11	1.00
22	4	3	4	4	2	4	4	4	4	4	4	11	0.91
23	4	3	4	4	4	4	4	4	4	4	4	11	1.00
24	4	3	4	4	4	4	4	4	4	4	4	11	1.00
25	3	3	4	4	4	4	4	4	3	4	4	11	1.00
26	4	3	4	4	4	4	4	4	3	4	4	11	1.00

Item	E1	E2	E3	E4	E5	E6	E7	E8	E9	E10	E11	Number of experts	I-CVI
27	4	3	4	4	4	4	4	4	4	4	4	11	1.00
28	4	3	3	4	1	4	4	4	3	4	4	11	0.91
29	4	3	4	4	1	4	4	4	4	4	4	11	0.91
30	4	3	4	4	4	4	4	4	4	4	4	11	1.00
31	4	2	4	4	4	4	4	4	3	4	4	11	0.91
32	4	3	4	4	1	4	4	4	3	4	4	11	0.91
33	4	3	4	4	4	4	4	4	3	4	4	11	1.00
34	4	3	4	4	1	4	4	4	4	4	4	11	0.91
35	4	4	4	4	3	4	4	4	2	4	4	11	0.91
36	4	4	4	4	3	4	4	4	2	4	4	11	0.91
37	4	2	4	4	4	4	4	4	3	4	4	11	0.91
38	4	4	4	4	4	4	4	4	4	4	4	11	1.00
39	4	3	4	4	3	4	4	3	4	4	4	11	1.00
												S-CVI/Ave = 0.95	

I-CVI = item content validity index; S-CVI, content validity index for the scale.

Table 2. Item-level content validity index for peripheral cannula insertion.

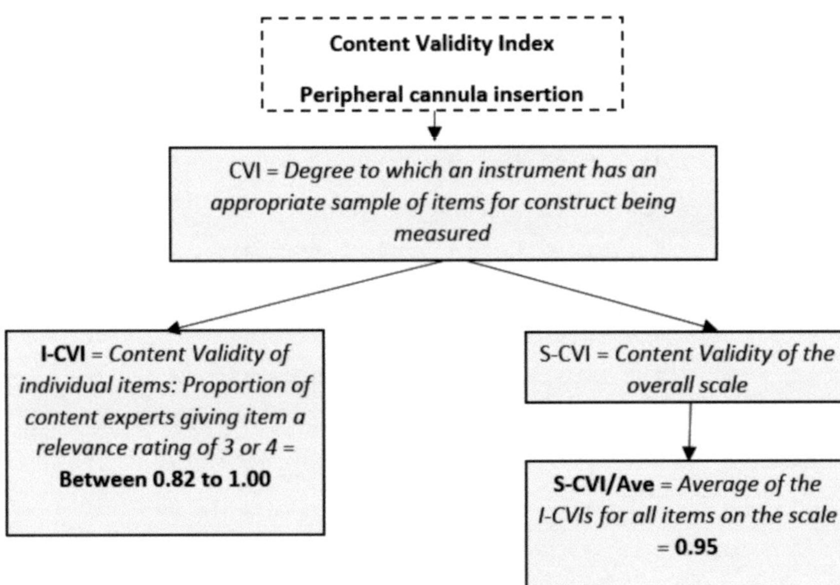

Figure 2. Elements of content validity index in peripheral cannula insertion check-list.

All I-CVI scores were summated to calculate S-CVI/Ave and then divided by the number of items: (0.82 + 0.82 + 0.91 + ... + 1.00)/39 = 0.95. All calculated results of S-CVI/Ave exceeded 0.90, which in combination with CVI (S-CVI) levels above 0.78 (**Table 2**) represent excellent content validity (**Table 3**) [19].

Essential nursing skills	Areas in nursing	Number of items	S-CVI/ave
Peripheral cannula insertion	Diagnostic/therapeutic essential nursing skills	39	0.95
Urinary catheterization: female	Elimination	54	0.95
Medication: injection of intravenous drugs	Medical management	28	0.94
Mouth care in unconscious patients	Personal hygiene	28	0.93
Insertion of a nasogastric tube	Nutrition	36	0.93
Suctioning the nasopharyngeal airway	Respiratory care	51	0.92

Table 3. Ranking of essential nursing skills from highest to lowest based on their content validity index average.

4. Discussion and conclusion

Methodological phases described in this pilot study could be considered and implemented when developing and establishing the checklist, which is designed to measure nursing students' performance during clinical skills assessment using OSCE. The purpose of developing a DOC score in the study was to represent the range of complexity in essential nursing skills and to identify criteria for further research in the CVI phase. Results of the CVI analysis demonstrated a good content validity (I-CVI and S-CVI/Ave) for the essential nursing skills that were included in the evaluation.

The benefits of using CVI for OSCE checklists have to be considered in terms of how it might undermine the essential nursing skill as a whole. For example, the calculated CVI for some items in a procedure might be calculated as lower than recommended. That in turn questions the need for the item within an essential nursing skill, and yet it is argued that every item in an essential nursing skill has a purpose. Eliminating those items with a low CVI could therefore be detrimental to the whole OSCE essential nursing skill and presents a challenge to nurse educators. On the other hand, CVI is widely used for developing different methodological researching tools [21–25].

Using OSCE in undergraduate nursing education offers a fresh approach for nurse educators in Slovenia and provides a new opportunity for determining nursing students' competency levels in simulated environment.

Findings from the CVI analysis are promising for developing OSCE checklist and are promising for further research using OSCE as an assessment modality.

Author details

Nino Fijačko[1]*, Zvonka Fekonja[1], Margaret Denny[1], Brian Sharvin[2], Majda Pajnkihar[1,3] and Gregor Štiglic[1,4]

*Address all correspondence to: nino.fijacko@um.si

1 Faculty of Health Sciences, University of Maribor, Maribor, Slovenia

2 School of Health Sciences, Waterford Institute of Technology, Waterford, Ireland

3 Faculty of Medicine, University of Maribor, Maribor, Slovenia

4 Faculty of Electrical Engineering and Computer Science, University of Maribor, Maribor, Slovenia

References

[1] Harden RM, Stevenson M, Downie WW, Wilson GM. Assessment of clinical competence using objective structured examination. British Medical Journal. 1975;**5955**:447–451

[2] Pegram A, Fordham-Clarke C. Implementing peer learning to prepare students for OSCEs. British Journal of Nursing. 2015;**24**:1060–1065. DOI: 10.12968/bjon.2015.24.21.1060

[3] Stunden A, Halcomb E, Jefferies D. Tools to reduce first year nursing students' anxiety levels prior to undergoing objective structured clinical assessment (OSCA) and how this impacts on the student's experience of their first clinical placement. Nurse Education Today. 2015;**35**:987–991.DOI: 10.1016/j.nedt.2015.04.014

[4] Harden RM. What is an OSCE? Medical Teacher. 1998;**10**:9–22

[5] Alinier G. Nursing students' and lecturers' perspectives of objective structured clinical examination incorporating simulation. Nurse Education Today. 2003;**23**:419–426

[6] McWilliam P, Botwinski C. Developing a successful nursing Objective Structured Clinical Examination. The Journal of Nursing Education. 2010;**49**:36–41. DOI: 10.3928/01484834-20090915-01

[7] Barry M, Noonan M, Bradshaw C, Murphy-Tighe S. An exploration of student midwives' experiences of the Objective Structured Clinical Examination assessment process. Nurse Education Today. 2012;**32**:690–694. DOI: 10.1016/j.nedt.2011.09.007

[8] Traynor M, Galanouli D. Have OSCEs come of age in nursing education? British Journal of Nursing. 2015;**24**:388–391. DOI: 10.12968/bjon.2015.24.7.388

[9] Mitchell ML, Jeffrey CA, Henderson A, Glover P, Nulty DD, Kelly MA, Groves M, Knight S. Using an Objective Structured Clinical Examination for Bachelor of Midwifery

students' preparation for practice. Women and Birth. 2014;**27**:108–113. DOI: 10.1016/j.wombi.2013.12.002

[10] Rushforth HE. Objective structured clinical examination (OSCE): Review of literature and implications for nursing education. Nurse Education Today. 2007;**27**:481–490

[11] Elliot DL, Fields SA, Keenen TL, Jaffe AC, Toffler WL. Use of a group objective structured clinical examination with first-year medical students. Academic Medicine. 1994;**69**:990–992

[12] Humphris GM, Kaney S. The objective structured video exam for assessment of communication skills. Medical Education. 2000;**34**:939–945

[13] Martin JA, Regehr G, Reznick R, MacRae H, Murnaghan J, Hutchison C, Brown M. Objective structured assessment of technical skill (OSATS) for surgical residents. British Journal of Surgery. 1997;**84**:273–278

[14] Simpson D, Lawrence S, Krogull S. Using standardized ambulatory teaching situations for faculty development. Teaching and Learning in Medicine. 1992;**4**:58–61

[15] Harden RM, Lilley P, Norman G. The Definitive Guide to the OSCE: The Objective Structured Clinical Examination as a Performance Assessment. 1st ed. Churchill Livingstone: Elsevier Health Sciences; 2015. p. 42

[16] Mårtensson G, Löfmark A. Implementation and student evaluation of clinical final examination in nursing education. Nurse Education Today. 2013;**33**:1563–1568. DOI: 10.1016/j.nedt.2013.01.003

[17] Miller B, Carr KC. Integrating standardized patients and objective structured clinical examinations into a nurse practitioner curriculum. The Journal for Nurse Practitioners. 2016;**12**:e201-e210

[18] Polit DF, Beck CT. The content validity index: Are you sure you know what's being reported? Critique and recommendations. Research in Nursing & Health. 2006;**29**:489–497. DOI: 10.1016/j.nurpra.2016.01.017

[19] Polit DF, Beck CT, Owen SV. Is the CVI an acceptable indicator of content validity? Appraisal and recommendations. Research in Nursing & Health. 2007;**30**:459–467

[20] Chumley HS. What does an OSCE checklist measure? Family Medicine. 2008;**40**:589–591

[21] Cooper S, Cant R, Porter J, Sellick K, Somers G, Kinsman L, Nestel D. Rating medical emergency teamwork performance: Development of the Team Emergency Assessment Measure (TEAM). Resuscitation. 2010;**81**:446–452. DOI: 10.1016/j.resuscitation.2009.11.027

[22] Beattie M, Shepherd A, Lauder W, Atherton I, Cowie J, Murphy DJ. Development and preliminary psychometric properties of the Care Experience Feedback Improvement Tool (CEFIT).BMJ Open. 2016;**6**:e010101. DOI: 10.1136/bmjopen-2015-010101

[23] Liaw SY, Scherpbier A, Klainin-Yobas P, Rethans JJ. Rescuing A Patient In Deteriorating Situations (RAPIDS): An evaluation tool for assessing simulation performance on clinical deterioration. Resuscitation. 2011;**82**:1434–1439. DOI: 10.1016/j.resuscitation.2011.06.008

[24] Hsu LL, Hsieh SI. Development and psychometric evaluation of the competency inventory for nursing students: A learning outcome perspective. Nurse Education Today. 2013;**33**:492–497. DOI: 10.1016/j.nedt.2012.05.028

[25] Ulfvarson J, Oxelmark L. Developing an assessment tool for intended learning outcomes in clinical practice for nursing students. Nurse Education Today. 2012;**32**:703–708. DOI: 10.1016/j.nedt.2011.09.010

Chapter 4

Comparing Students' Self-Assessment with Teachers' Assessment of Clinical Skills Using an Objective Structured Clinical Examination (OSCE)

Zvonka Fekonja, Jasmina Nerat, Vida Gönc,
Milena Pišlar, Margaret Denny and
Klavdija Čuček Trifkovič

Additional information is available at the end of the chapter

http://dx.doi.org/10.5772/67956

Abstract

Evaluation of clinical skills is a demanding and complex process and is dependent on many complex factors, such as teaching and learning approaches, simulated learning, and psychometrically validated assessment tools. Therefore, it is imperative that adequate strategies and methods are employed to evaluate the success of a nursing care activity. One such strategy in the field of nursing care is the application of objective structured clinical examination (OSCE) of a nursing activity. The purpose of this article is to highlight the importance of evaluating nursing activities in a simulated clinical environment with OSCE to determine synchronicity of the teacher and student assessment. A cross-sectional study was carried out, in which we compared the evaluation of nursing activity by the teacher and the 51 students. Summative content analysis was used to analyze open-ended questions about possible improvement of performed nursing activity. The data showed a large discrepancy (81.9%) in evaluating nursing activity between the teacher and the student. The synchronicity between the teacher and student assessment modality occurred only in 18%. Students were mostly less successful in their assessment of competence with knowledge about carrying out interventions (36.5%), preparing for interventions (24.3%), and infection control (14.4%). Clinical skills acquisition remains an essential element of a student nurse's development, as competence in nursing skills is essential to patient safety. Simulation is viewed as an increasingly popular approach to the teaching and assessing of clinical skills. The process of evaluating nursing activity demands the usage of objective instruments that require objectivity, fairness, impartiality, and comprehension. The use of OSCE is one such method of promoting reliable and valid assessments in nursing skills.

Keywords: nursing care activities, assessment, OSCE, teacher, student

1. Introduction

Nursing is a discipline based on clinical practice–based interventions [1] with the purpose of nursing development and adjusting to needs of contemporary society [2]. The study of nursing care must prepare students to carry out and accept professional responsibility in a changing clinical environment [3–5]. Only in a clinical environment does a nurse's knowledge become most evident [6]. Because of the importance of clinical training, appropriate strategies for clinical assessment must be sought, with the purpose of specifying a success rate of clinical training [7]. Such strategies are important for evaluating the quality of teaching and learning processes [8], identifying student's weaknesses, increasing their motivation for competence achievement, and helping teachers to assess their work [9–12]. Knowledge evaluation is a time intensive and complicated process, leaning mostly on teacher's subjective judgment. In addition, students identify they are not satisfied with current methods and results of assessment [7, 13, 14].

Simulated learning using objective structured clinical examination (OSCE) has emerged as an alternative teaching method to assist students in acquiring clinical skills competency because it attempts to replicate a real-life situation in a simulated environment [15, 16]. There is a current trend in nursing education to use OSCE to assess and examine clinical competence [16, 17] within this simulated setting. The OSCE was originally designed for the medical profession [18] but has been modified and applied in nursing education, providing means to assess competence in a simulated environment without posing a risk to patient safety [16, 19]. A number of studies using various research designs including qualitative [20, 21], quantitative [22], and mixed methods [23, 24] have all reported positive results from using OSCE as a teaching methodology [16].

Objective structured clinical examination is a versatile multipurpose assessment tool that can be used to evaluate the nursing care that students deliver to patients in a clinical setting [25]. It is used in a planned and structured manner with a clear emphasis on objectivity [26]. Additionally, as an assessment tool, it uses a task analysis of general clinical skills [27] specific to the student's program and year of study and as stated previously is usually carried out in a simulated environments [28, 29]. Contrary to traditional assessment modalities, OSCE evaluates areas that are most critical to nursing competence, for example, blood pressure, pulse, respiration, communication skills, and various other nursing interventions [25] in a simulated work environment [30]. The OSCE has for a long time been recognized as a formal assessment method in medical education [31] and is now more frequently used as an assessment method in nursing [32, 33]. It is argued that despite the rhetoric of a student-centered approach, education remains wedded to conventional teaching and learning approaches, which fail to engage with the individual and unwittingly silence the individual's voice [34, 35]. Therefore, it is imperative that more contemporary student-centered approaches to teaching and learning are incorporated in nursing assessment.

The OSCE assessment tool was introduced to the University of Maribor Faculty of Health Sciences to examine performance of various clinical skills in a simulated clinical environment. The course unit of study was "Nursing Care in academic year 2015/2016" (first year

http://dx.doi.org/10.5772/67956

students of nursing care). Standardized assessment checklists were evaluated together with the teacher's assessment of clinical training success. Students were encouraged to reflect on various nursing case scenarios in order to recognize mistakes and ensure competent practice. Simulation as a teaching method allows for multiple learning objectives to be taught in a realistic clinical environment without causing harm to patients and can provide 'microworlds' whereby important interactions between patients, doctors, nurses, and other health professionals can be highlighted, illustrated, explained, and replayed [16, 36].

Emphasis was placed on recognizing the mistakes made by both students and teacher when carrying out various nursing care skills and on the aspects of practice they did. The following research questions were posed:

1. Is there consensus between student and teacher evaluations when assessing nursing practice using an OSCE?
2. Does a student assessed with OSCE method recognize mistakes made when carrying out various nursing care skills?
3. Can the student critically evaluate the performed nursing care activity in concordance with teacher's evaluations?

2. Methodology

2.1. Design

To answer the research questions, a cross sectional observational research study was used. Nursing students performed care activities within an OSCE situation and then assessed their own performance. The nursing care was also independently assessed by a teacher. In this study, we compared these assessments. To explore this, we conducted an analysis of open-ended question about possible improvements of nursing care activity using summative content analysis.

2.2. Setting and participants

An initial available sample of 51 participants was recruited from a cohort of first-year B.Sc. general nursing students using an available sampling approach. Available sampling involves taking a sample of what one would call typical, normal, or average for a particular phenomenon under study [37]. All students were recruited through purposive sampling. The student successfully completed training in the clinical skills laboratory for nursing care of an adult patient and also successfully passed mid-term assessment. Participants were all first year nursing students who had completed the same clinical skills training course in the 1st degree study program of Nursing Care. The majority of participants (46.90%) were female. The response rate was 56% (n = 52). This means that more than half of the students completed the OSCE and wrote a reflective piece. Assessment was carried out by higher education teachers of nursing care in January 2016. Students had to meet the following inclusion criteria: (1) active participation at laboratory clinical skills in a simulated clinical environment (150 hours), (2) student's assessment based on OSCE assessment paper, (3) student's reflective writing after completing the nursing care activity, and (4) written self-evaluation.

2.3. Ethical considerations

The study complied with ethical procedures of research, the Declaration of Helsinki, provisions of the Oviedo Convention and Code of Ethics for nurses and medical technicians from Slovenia [38], which was adhered here throughout the process. Research participants' anonymity was assured by numerical coding of their written self-evaluation sheet, so that the participants could not be identified from the information. Data collection took place in classroom settings, and participation in the research was completely voluntary. The research team was the only people who had access to the data, and the data were stored on a computer that was password protected.

2.4. Data collection

Students' practical work at the course unit Nursing Care was assessed with objective structured clinical examination checklist OSCE, which consisted of 42 clinical skills. The checklist was composed by teachers, which perform training for students in the clinical skills laboratory. Each checklist of simulated interventions consisted of a series of performance-based observations and rated students' performance as completed accurately; inaccurately or not completed. Students were acquainted with the method of evaluation for their clinical skills competence, and they also had the opportunity to view the assessment checklist items. All OSCE assessors had worked previously with the students in the clinical skills laboratory. An independent evaluator (a teacher who didn't participate in the training process) assessed the students during the performance of the nursing care activity by observing and filling out the assessment checklists. Using OSCE, 42 nursing care activities were evaluated. After performing the nursing intervention, the students had approximately 10 min to evaluate their nursing care activity using an unstructured method of reflection with the purpose of analyzing mistakes and endeavoring to improve future practice of such skills and prevent student from being awarded a fail grade. To assist the critical reflection process, students were posed a question: *What could you have improved during carried out intervention or would you improve something?*

2.5. Data analysis

The first and last author transcribed the students' reflective writing (after 1 month of the evaluation process). The transcripts were then analyzed and coded by two authors (ZF & KČT) using descriptive statistics and summative content analysis [39] for analysis of the open-ended question. This approach contains a quantitative element, because the results show in the proportions of how many times some words are repeated or a response depending on the particular subject of research. Summative content analysis includes counting and comparing

http://dx.doi.org/10.5772/67956

keywords and content with the interpretation of the meaning of these [39]. In the first step, the reflective sheets were read carefully, trying to obtain a sense of the entire contents [39, 40] and then to derive topics. We highlight the exact word from the text, which covered the main idea or concept. The incidence of identified keyword and concepts were then calculated and presented in percentages. This method was chosen as there was a large quantity of data [40] and using this approach enabled the opportunity to quantify words or content and subsequent data interpretation.

3. Results

Answers to the open question were categorized in six themes (see **Table 1**) and organized after occurrence—from most frequent to less frequent repetition.

The analysis of clinical skills' evaluation (performing a nursing care activity) showed that students were least successful at themes of "Knowledge needed for carried out interventions (159 [36.5%])" that contained theoretical and practical knowledge needed for the successful performance of an intervention. Themes of category "Treatment after intervention" were assessed as less successful from student's and teacher's assessment viewpoint (15 [3.4%]).

Student's and teacher's assessments were in harmony in 18.1%, regarding all items of the assessment papers. In 81.9%, the assessments were not in harmony (**Table 2**).

Theme	Number of items	Percentage (%)	Meaning
Knowledge needed for carried out interventions	159	36.5	Theoretical and practical knowledge
Preparation for intervention	106	24.3	Assuring privacy, condition evaluation, preparation of the room and accessories
Infections treatment	63	14.4	Disinfection of material, accessories and hands, preventives, recycling
Safety assurance	51	11.6	Placement of safety protectors and buzzer by the bed, comparison of identity and doctor's requirements, marking of material
Communication skills	43	9.8	Explanation of purpose, goal and course of care intervention, obtaining of an agreement, passing future instructions
Treatment after intervention	15	3.4	Fixing up the patient, arranging of material and of the room, documenting
Total	435	100	

Table 1. Content analysis and occurring themes.

Harmony	Number	Percentage (%)
Yes	79	18.1
No	357	81.9
Total	436	100

Table 2. Harmony of the student's and teacher's assessment.

Most discrepancies at evaluation were noted in items of "Knowledge needed for carried out interventions," where discrepancy between the student's and teacher's assessment was 37%. Least discrepancies were noted at items of "Treatment after interventions," 3.5% (**Table 3**).

Theme	Total number of items	Percentage (%)	Student's grade N (%)		Teacher's grade N (%)	
Preparation for intervention	88	24.3	24	19.7	64	26.6
Infection management	48	13.2	23	18.8	25	10.4
Communication skills	38	10.5	17	13.9	21	8.8
Safety assurance	43	11.8	13	10.6	30	12.5
Knowledge needed for carried out interventions	134	37.0	41	33.6	93	38.7
Treatment after intervention	13	3.5	5	4.0	8	3.3
Total	362	100	122	100	240	100

Table 3. Discrepancy of the student's and teacher's assessment regarding themes.

4. Discussion

For assessment of a nursing care activity, we sought approaches that help teachers objectively evaluate student's knowledge. One of such instrument for evaluation of theoretical knowledge and performance of nursing care activity is the OSCE [41]. In the research carried out on 51 first-year nursing care students, we wanted to find out differences in assessment of a nursing care activity between a student and a teacher in a simulated environment. The data identified a big discrepancy (81.9%) in the evaluation of nursing care. Harmony between the teacher and student was present only in 18% of the data. On completion of the activity, students had to write their reflection about performance and answer questions on possible improvements. In this process, they showed a lack of criticism and in-depth performance insight. This supported other literature [25] as the most critical assessment areas: communication skills and ability to manage patient's inappropriate behavior. In our research, we found out that a student was least successful in the knowledge area of intervention performance, preparation for intervention, and infection management. Results indicate that students lacked self-criticism and lack of theoretical knowledge. The reference [42] states that objective methods for assessment are an appropriate alternative to traditional knowledge assessment forms. These methods are even more effective because of instant feedback of students and teachers [43]. As in previous studies [44, 45], the methods of objective assessment requires a lot of time, many teachers, and financial investment, although this should be balanced with greater satisfaction to students and teachers.

4.1. Limitations of this study

Our research has some limitations that require careful consideration. Because of a small sample, generalization is less reliable. Students were not assessed using exactly the same interventions. They chose interventions randomly, and they were not the same level of difficulty. Audio and video recording as a feedback method on their own performance for recognizing mistakes was not assessed. A structured reflective model was not used as students wrote their reflection based on questions posed by the teacher. Finally, the assessment was performed by one teacher; therefore, adequate tests of objectivity cannot be assured.

5. Implications for nursing education

OSCE is an assessment technique in which students perform nursing interventions under a variety of simulated conditions. Through the assessment of students, performance on the same skill and of the same place, the equity, and the objectivity to the students are enhanced. The introduction of a student self-assessment checklist contributed to a reflection of their own performance of each step of the skill before evaluation with OSCE and prompt identification of student's strengths and weaknesses during exercise of skills performance. Using the OSCE as an assessment method that is based on real scenarios increased the confidence of student.

6. Conclusion

There has been increased attention over the past decades on the use of objective structured clinical examination systems as a training and assessment tool. OSCE mainly assesses basic knowledge and technical performance of an activity. It is harder to assess the ability of critical thinking, interacting communication skills, experiencing, student's expectations and skills, in order to treat a patient like a whole. The use of new assessment systems is limited and one-sided; therefore, a richer combination of assessment systems is required. In pursuing clinical competence in nursing students' clinical skills, nursing teachers have to endeavor to find new ways to assess and examine these essential skills that are necessary for patient safety and care. Future studies should include a larger sample of students, and the use of a reflective model to capture student perception of learning is recommended.

Author details

Zvonka Fekonja*, Jasmina Nerat, Vida Gönc, Milena Pišlar, Margaret Denny and Klavdija Čuček Trifkovič

*Address all correspondence to: zvonka.fekonja@um.si

Faculty of Health Sciences, Institute for Nursing Care, University of Maribor, Maribor, Slovenia

References

[1] Henderson A., Tyler S. Facilitating learning in clinical practice: Evaluation of a trial of a supervisor of clinical education role. Nurse Educ Pract 2011;**11**(5):188–92. DOI: 10.1016/j.nepr.2011.01.003.

[2] Farzianpour F., Monzavi A., Yassini E. Evaluating the quality of education at dentistry School of Tehran University of medical sciences. Dent Res J (Isfahan) 2011;**8**(2):71–9.

[3] Liang L. The gap between evidence and practice. Health Aff 2007;**26**(2):w119–21. DOI: 10.1377/hlthaff.26.2.w119.

[4] Butler M.P., Cassidy I., Quillinan B., Fahy A., Bradshaw C., Tuohy D., O'Connor M., Mc Namara M.C., Egan G. Competency assessment methods – Tool and processes: A survey of nurse preceptors in Ireland. Nurse Educ Pract 2011;**11**(5):298–303. DOI: 10.1016/j.nepr.2011.01.006.

[5] Chiang V.C., Chan S.S. An evaluation of advanced simulation in nursing: A mixed-method study. Collegian 2014;**21**(4):257–65.

[6] Mansoorian M.R., Hosseiny M.S., Khosravan S., Alami A., Alaviani M. Comparing the effects of objective structured assessment of technical skills (OSATS) and traditional method on learning of students. Nurs Midwifery Stud 2015;**4**(2):e27714. DOI: 10.17795/nmsjournal27714.

[7] Noohi E., Motesadi M., Haghdoost A. Clinical teachers' viewpoints towards objective structured clinical examination in Kerman University of Medical Science. Iran J Med Educ 2008;**8**(1):113–20.

[8] Iqbal M., Khizar B., Zaidi Z. Revising an objective structured clinical examination in a resource-limited Pakistani Medical School. Educ Health (Abingdon) 2009;**22**(1):209.

[9] Joyce B. Developing an Assessment System Facilitator's Guide. Accreditation Council for Graduate Medical Education 2006;**1**:15–17.

[10] Epstein R.M. Assessment in medical education. N Engl J Med 2007;**256**(4):387–96. DOI: 10.1056/NEJMra054784.

[11] Aronson L., Niehaus B., Hill-Sakurai L., Lai C., O'Sullivan P.S. A comparison of two methods of teaching reflective ability in year 3 medical students. Med Educ 2012;**46**(8):807–14. DOI: 10.1111/j.1365-2923.2012.04299.x.

[12] Fernández-Sola C., Granero-Molina J., Márquez-Membrive J., Aguilera-Manrique G., Castro-Sánchez A.M. Implementation of the new clinical practice training model in Andalusia: A qualitative evaluation of the nursing and physiotherapy degrees. Enferm Clin 2014;**24**(2):136–41. DOI: 10.1016/j.enfcli.2013.09.004.

[13] Wilkinson T.J., Frampton C.M. Comprehensive undergraduate medical assessments improve prediction of clinical performance. Med Educ 2004;**38**(10):1111–6. DOI: 10.1111/j.1365-2929.2004.01962.x.

[14] Cheater F.M., Baker R., Reddish S., Spiers N., Wailoo A., Gillies C., Robertson N., Cawood C. Cluster randomized controlled trial of the effectiveness of audit and feedback and educational outreach on improving nursing practice and patient outcomes. Med Care 2006;**44**(6):542–51. DOI: 10.1097/01.mlr.0000215919.89893.8a.

[15] Decker S., Sportsman S., Puetz L., Billings L. The evolution of simulation and its contribution to competency. J Contin Educ Nurs 2008;**39**(2):74–80.

[16] Sharvin B. Theory-Practice Integration for Clinical Skills Competence among Undergraduate Nursing Students in Ireland: A Mixed Method Study [thesis] 2016. Thesis submitted to the University of Derby for award of Doctor of Education.

[17] Meechan R., Jones H., Valler-Jones T. Students' perspectives on their skills acquisition and confidence. Br J Nurs 2011;**20**(7):445–50. DOI: 10.12968/bjon.2011.20.7.445.

[18] Harden R.M., Gleeson F.A. Assessment of clinical competence using an objective structured clinical examination (OSCE). Med Educ 1979;**13**:41–54. DOI: 10.1111/j.1365-2923.1979.tb00918.x.

[19] Cant R., McKenna L., Cooper S. Assessing preregistration nursing students' clinical competence: A systematic review of objective measures. Int J Nurs Pract 2013;**19**(2):163–76. DOI: 10.1111/ijn.12053.

[20] Morgan D.L. Paradigms lost and pragmatism regained: Methodological implications of combining qualitative and quantitative methods. J Mixed Methods Res 2007;**1**(1):48–76. DOI: 10.1177/2345678906292462.

[21] Houghton C.E., Casey D., Shaw D., Murphy K. Students' experiences of implementing clinical skills in the real world of practice. J Clin Nurs 2013;**22**(13–14):1961–9. DOI: 10.1111/jocn.12014.

[22] Nevin M., Neill F., Mulkerrins J. Preparing the nursing student for internship in a pre-registration nursing program: Developing a problem based approach with the use of high fidelity simulation equipment. Nurse Educ Pract 2014;**14**(2):154–9. DOI: 10.1016/j.nepr.2013.07.008.

[23] McCaughey C.S., Traynor M.K. The role of simulation in nurse education. Nurse Educ Today 2010;**30**(8):827–32. DOI: 10.1016/j.nedt.2010.03.005.

[24] Hope A., Garside J., Prescott S. Rethinking theory and practice: Pre-registration student nurses experiences of simulation teaching and learning in the acquisition of clinical skills in preparation for practice. Nurse Educ Today 2011;**31**(7):711–5. DOI: 10.1016/j.nedt.2010.12.011.

[25] Zayyan M. Objective structured clinical examination: The assessment of choice. Oman Med J 2011;**26**(4):219–22. DOI: 10.5001/omj.2011.55.

[26] Harden R.M. What is an OSCE?. Med Teach 1988;**10**(1):19–22. DOI: 10.3109/01421598809019321.

[27] Ward H., Willis A. Assessing advanced clinical practice skills. Prim Health Care 2006;**16**(3):22–4. DOI: 10.7748/phc.16.3.22.s23.

[28] Merriman C., Westcott L. Succeed in OSCEs and Practical Exams: An Essential Guide for nurses 2010. 1st ed. Maidenhead: McGraw-Hill Education.

[29] Fidment S. The objective structured clinical exam (OSCE): A qualitative study exploring the healthcare student's experience. Stud Engagem Exp J 2012;**1**(1):1–11. DOI: 10.7190/seej.v1i1.37.

[30] Mitchell M.L., Henderson A., Groves M., Dalton M., Nulty D. The objective structured clinical examination (OSCE): Optimising its value in the undergraduate nursing curriculum. Nurse Educ Today 2009;**29**(4):398–404. DOI: 10.1016/j.nedt.2008.10.007.

[31] Ward H., Barratt J. Assessment of nurse practitioner advanced clinical practice skills: Using the objective structured clinical examination (OSCE). Prim Health Care 2005;**15**(10):37–41. DOI: 10.7748/phc2005.12.15.10.37.c563.

[32] Wessel J., Williams R., Finch E., Gémus M. Reliability and validity of an objective structured clinical examination for physical therapy students. J Allied Health 2003;**32**(4):266–9.

[33] Bartfay W.J., Rombough R., Howse E., Leblanc R. Evaluation. The OSCE approach in nursing education. Can Nurse 2004;**100**(3):18–23.

[34] Denny M., Redmond-Stokes O., Wells J., Weber E., O'Sullivan K., Taylor, M. The learning experience: A new approach to optimise student learning. In: Callara E.. editor. Nursing Education Challenges in the 21st Century 2008. 1st ed. New York: Nova Science Publisher. pp. 23–48.

[35] Denny M., Weber E.F., Wells J., Stokes O.R., Lane P., Denieffe S. Matching purpose with practice: Revolutionising nurse education with mita. Nurse Educ Today 2008;**28**(1):100–7. DOI: 10.1016/j.nedt.2007.03.004.

[36] Valler-Jones T., Meechan R., Jones H. Simulated practice—a panacea for health education?. Br J Nurs 2011;**20**(10):628–31. DOI: 10.12968/bjon.2011.20.10.628.

[37] Heppner P., Kivlingham D.M., Wampold B.E. Research Design in Counseling 1992. Pacific Grove, CA: Brooks/Cole.

[38] Ovijač D., Velepič M., Adamič M., Eder J., et al. Kodeks etike v zdravstveni negi in oskrbi Slovenije. Ljubljana: Zbornica zdravstvene in babiške nege – Zveza strokovnih društev medicinskih sester, babic in zdravstvenih tehnikov Slovenije 2014.

[39] Hsieh H.F., Shannon S.E. Three approaches to qualitative content analysis. Qual Health Res 2005;**15**(9):1277–88. DOI: 10.1177/1049732305276687.

[40] Elo S., Kyngäs H. The qualitative content analysis process. J Adv Nurs 2008;**62**(1):107–15. DOI: 10.1111/j.1365-2648.2007.04569.x.

[41] Stunden A., Halcomb E., Jefferies D. Tools to reduce first year nursing students' anxiety levels prior to undergoing objective structured clinical assessment (OSCA) and how this impacts on the student's experience of their first clinical placement. Nurse Educ Today 2015;**35**(9):987–91. DOI: 10.1016/j.nedt.2015.04.014.

[42] Akhtar-Danesh N., Valaitis R., O'Mara L., Austin P., Munroe V. Viewpoints about collaboration between primary care and public health in Canada. BMC Health Serv Res 2013;**13**:311. DOI: 10.1186/1472-6963-13-311.

[43] Rushforth H.E. Objective structured clinical examination (OSCE): review of literature and implications for nursing education. Nurse Educ Today 2007;**27**(5):481–90. DOI: 10.1016/j.nedt.2006.08.009.

[44] Berkenstadt H., Ziv A., Gafni N., Sidi A. Incorporating simulation-based objective structured clinical examination into the Israeli National Board Examination in Anesthesiology. Anesth Analg 2006;**102**(3):853–8. DOI: 10.1213/01.ane.0000194934.34552.ab.

[45] AbdiShahshahani M., Ehsanpour S., Yamani N., Kohan S. The evaluation of reproductive health PhD program in Iran: The input indicators analysis. Iran J Nurs Midwifery Res 2014;**19**(6):620–8.

Chapter 5

Assessment of Clinical Nursing Competencies: Literature Review

Nataša Mlinar Reljić, Mateja Lorber,
Dominika Vrbnjak, Brian Sharvin and Maja Strauss

Additional information is available at the end of the chapter

http://dx.doi.org/10.5772/67362

Abstract

Introduction: In Slovene nursing higher education, there is a lack of empirical evidence to support the choice of tolls for assessment of clinical skills and competencies. This literature review aims to critically discuss identified methods of clinical nursing skills assessment and competencies currently used in nursing higher education in other countries.

Methods: An electronic data base search was conducted using Medline, CINAHL, and PubMed. The search was limited to empirical research published within the previous 5 years. Full-text available articles published in peer-reviewed journals and written in English were included. The Mixed Methods Appraisal Tool (MMAT) was used to appraise and describe the methodological quality. The synthesis of the results was reported narratively.

Results: From 160 identified records, 12 studies were retained based on the inclusion and exclusion criteria. A number of approaches are currently being used and include a variety of assessment tools, objective structured clinical examinations (OSCEs), and complex assessment approaches.

Discussion and conclusion: Results present an overview of current clinical assessment in the clinical environment and in the clinical skills laboratories (CSLs). There is a need to develop a holistic approach to clinical skills competency assessment with a reasonable level of validity and reliability.

Keywords: assessment, clinical skill, clinical competence, nursing competencies

1. Introduction

Nursing students have to develop clinical knowledge, skills, and attitudes for professional practice, and nursing educators have to assess and evaluate students' core skills readiness for clinical practice [1], and the assessment should be a real indicator of knowledge [2]. Assessment in clinical practice can either be formative or summative [3], with the formative often used to discuss and analyze students' performance [4] and the summative examining practical performance in the clinical or simulation environment [5]. Both methods should ensure that the criteria for assessment reference the intended learning outcomes [6].

Three approaches to assessment of assessing nursing students' nursing competencies were identified from the literature and include observation methods [1, 7], self-perception methods [8] and methods combining both approaches [9]. Of these methods, observation of student performance and the use of skills checklists appear to be the most common [10, 11]. This can be done either by direct observation in the clinical environment [7, 12] or by observing the student in the clinical skills laboratory (CLS) using scenarios and clinical skills checklists to measure performance [1]. Other multimethod approaches are used and include clinical portfolio evaluation [13], along with critical incident reports, case-based assessment, peer assessment [9], and reflection [14]. Reflection is important because nurses need to think critically and reflection develops responsibility in clinical practice [15].

The last decade has seen the emergence of new measurement tools being developed and tested for validity and reliability [16]. These include the objective structured clinical examinations (OSCEs) [1] that have numerous advantages over other observation tools [17], such as the development of student's self-confidence [18], the grounding of more expressive learning [19], and the assessment of not only psychomotor skills but also allows for the assessment of knowledge and attitudes [20]. The OSCE, however, is not the only assessment tool used in nursing education. There are numbers of different scales for assessing student's competencies and psychometric properties [21–23]. This literature reviews, therefore, set out to identify and critically analyze current methods of clinical nursing skills assessment and competencies used in nursing higher education in other countries with regard to developing a comprehensive and effective method for assessing clinical competency in Slovene nursing higher education.

1.1. Aim

The aim of this literature review is to identify methods of clinical nursing skills assessment and competencies currently used in nursing higher education in other countries.

2. Methods

2.1. Eligibility criteria

Studies were included if they met the following inclusion criteria: empirical research primarily focused on methods of clinical nursing skills and competencies assessment and their reliability and validity, full-text available articles published in peer-reviewed journals and written in English, published between 2010 and 2016. Exclusion criteria were systematic review articles, assessment of clinical nursing skills in vocational training, assessment of special clinical nursing skills, editorial and commentary pieces, and all other literature not meeting the inclusion criteria.

2.2. Search strategy and study identification

Three electronic databases were searched for relevant literature: Medline, CINAHL, and PubMed. Key word combinations that were used included competency, competence, clinical competency, clinical competencies, clinical skill, clinical competence, professional competence, competency based education, assessment, measuring, measurement, test, scale, standards, validity, reliability, generalizability, and nursing student. Literature published within the last 5 years was searched due to the contemporary interest in clinical skills and competencies assessment in nursing.

2.3. Study selection and extraction

Identified references were merged with reference software EndNote, and duplicates were removed. The titles and abstracts of the identified results were then assessed for eligibility criteria by two of the authors (DV, ML). Studies not relevant to this review were removed. After retrieval of the full text, two of the authors (DV, ML) independently screened the studies and made decisions concerning final inclusion of the studies. A further two reviewers were then consulted (NMR, MS). Disagreements were solved by discussion. Data were extracted by predefined criteria, which included source, country, objectives, methods, and main findings.

2.4. Assessment of study quality

The Mixed Methods Appraisal Tool (MMAT) was used for assessing their quality. The tool is useful for appraising quantitative, qualitative, and mixed methods studies [24]. Methodological quality criteria are scored on a nominal scale. The tool includes two screening questions and four criteria for qualitative studies, quantitative randomized controlled trials, quantitative nonrandomized studies, quantitative descriptive studies, and three criteria for mixed methods. The score is based on the number of criteria met divided by four (from one criteria met—25% to all criteria met—100%) [24]. Each study was checked for quality by one author (NMR) and then rechecked by two other authors (ML, MS). Disagreements were solved by discussion until consensus was reached.

2.5. Data synthesis

A convergent qualitative synthesis design was selected and results from the identified studies were transformed into qualitative findings [25], using a narrative synthesis as described by Harrison et al. [26] and Dixon-Woods et al. [27]. This approach was selected as studies were heterogeneous.

3. Results

3.1. Study selection and its characteristics

The search revealed a total of 160 records. **Figure 1** provides a flow diagram of the literature selection process.

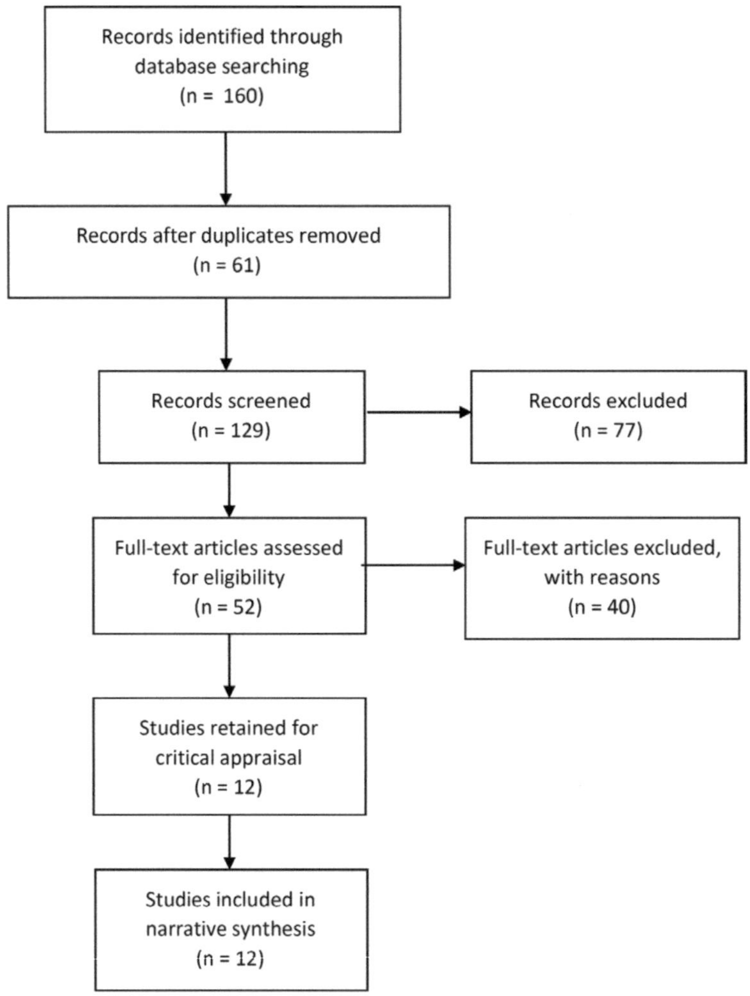

Figure 1. Flow diagram of literature selection.

The flow diagram (**Figure 1**) shows that after removing duplicates, 129 records were screened by title and abstract for their relevance, leading to the exclusion of 77 records. The remaining 52 full texts were assessed for eligibility. Critical reading of the full text led to 12 studies being retained for inclusion in the review.

3.2. Methodological quality of studies

The selected studies were conducted in Australia, Sweden, Iran, Canada, Ireland, Spain, Pakistan, and Taiwan. The studies have utilized different study designs, and a number of different methods were identified including a variety of assessment tools, OSCE, complex approaches, and others. There are presented selected studies objectives, design, main findings, and the MMAT score in **Table 1**.

Table 1 provides a detailed description of the individual studies included in the review. There are five columns in the table. The first column provides details of the source and origin of the study and are presented in alphabetical order. The second and third columns list the key objectives and the research design. The main findings are presented in the fourth column, and the final column lists the MMAT score.

Source and country	Objectives	Design	Main findings	MMAT
Athlin et al. [28] Sweden	To describe the development and evaluation of a model for a National Clinical Final Examination in the bachelor nursing education.	Collaborative project between four universities and adjunctive healthcare areas supplying clinical placements using the Delphi technique and literature review followed by evaluation.73 students included in theoretical test and 68 students included in bedside test.	• Theoretical test: problem-solving character, consists of two patient cases describing realistic situations in medical, surgical, or geriatric care in which the patient is followed throughout the care trajectory; the template of criteria for each case. • Bedside test: student is taking care for one patient (unknown to the students), while being observed by "an observing nurse" who is using an assessment tool: (1) assessment of needs and problems, analyzes, and planning, (2) implementation and evaluation of nursing activities and (3) reflections and final judgment. • Evaluation of a value, relevance and usability of the model. • Model was highly appreciated, and its relevance, usability, and validity considered as quite good for the assessment of nursing students' clinical competence at the final stage of their education, especially as not only focusing on assessment of technical skills. • Several deficiencies, needs further evaluation.	75%
Hengameh et al. [29] Iran	To compare the effect of applying direct observation procedural skills and routine	Randomized clinical trial. Nursing students included.	• Routine evaluation method: a subjective judgment of an instructor about general skills of the	100%

Source and country	Objectives	Design	Main findings	MMAT
	evaluation method on clinical skills of nursing students.		student during their clinical course hence the scoring. • Direct observation procedural skills: clinical activities evaluated based on direct observation using the checklists. • Evaluation in control group: in one stage by routine. • Evaluation in intervention group: (a) first stage test: (observation of the skills for 15 min and giving feedback for 5 min), (b) second stage test: repeating the first test after two weeks (emphasis on providing feedback on the students' strength and weakness), third stage test: repeating the first stage test after four weeks and giving the final scores to the student. • Final evaluation: prepared checklist. • No significant difference observed between the two groups in terms of demographic variables ($p > 0.05$). • A significant difference observed between intervention and control scores ($p = 0.000$). • Application of direct observation of procedural skills has improved clinical skills of the students significantly.	
Hsu and Hsieh [21] Taiwan	To develop a competency inventory to measure learning outcomes of baccalaureate nursing students and to test its psychometric properties.	Cross-sectional survey.599 nursing students included.	• Instrument measuring six factors. • Ethics and accountability were found to be the most important factor	75%

Source and country	Objectives	Design	Main findings	MMAT
			contributing to nursing student's competencies. • Satisfactory psychometric properties. • Useful instrument for measuring learning outcomes of nursing student.	
Iglesias-Parra et al. [30]Spain	To develop an evaluation system of clinical competencies for the practicum of nursing students based on the Nursing Interventions Classification (NIC).	Psychometric validation study: the first two phases addressed definition and content validation, and the third phase consisted of a cross-sectional study for analyzing reliability. The population of undergraduate nursing students and clinical tutors.	• Competencies were designed for second-year clinical placement, and using the same methodology, 18 additional interventions were identified to describe more clinical competencies to be achieved in the third year, reaching a total of 91 interventions. • A competency system for the nursing practicum, structured on the NIC, was found to be a reliable method for assessing and evaluating clinical competencies. • Further evaluations in other contexts are needed. • A tool based on the NIC is otherwise used for competency assessment in combination with a portfolio that includes a reflexive diary through a blog and objective structured clinical examinations.	100%
Imanipour and Jalili [31]Iran	To develop a comprehensive assessment system for nursing students in their critical care rotation based on a programmatic approach.	Development in three phases followed by assessment: determination of the educational objectives based on the nursing curriculum; identification of a list of appropriate assessment methods, selection; determination of a content validity.38 bachelor nursing students included.	• All items of the assessment system had a high CVR and CVI ranged. • The findings showed that 87.5% of the instructors and 89.47% of students believed that the new assessment system had a positive impact on learning. • A programmatic approach should be used	75%

Source and country	Objectives	Design	Main findings	MMAT
			for effective evaluation of clinical performance of nursing students in critical care settings because of high validity and reliability, multidimensionality, positive educational impact, and acceptability.	
Khan et al. [14] Pakistan	To identify nursing students' perceptions about the effectiveness of utilized teaching and learning strategies of clinical education, in improving students' knowledge, skills, and attitudes.	A descriptive cross-sectional study design using both qualitative and quantitative approaches.74 nursing students included.	• The findings revealed that the demonstration was the most effective strategy for improving students' skills; reflection, for improving attitudes; and problem-based learning and concept map for improving their knowledge. • Students' responses to open-ended questions confirmed the effectiveness of these strategies in improving their learning outcomes. • Identified perceptions about the effectiveness of the utilized teaching and learning strategies from students' point of view. • Problem-based learning and concept map were both viewed as very effective teaching and learning strategies for the development of students' knowledge, whereas the demonstration was perceived as an effective strategy for the development of their skills. • Reflection was felt to be more effective in the development of students' knowledge and for bringing about positive changes in attitudes.	50%
Levett-Jones et al. [32] Australia	To describe the design, implementation, and evaluation of the SOAP, a model used to assess third-year	Evaluation of Structured Observation and Assessment of Practice (SOAP) using quantitative and qualitative	• Four components showed acceptable factor loadings and that together accounted for	75%

Source and country	Objectives	Design	Main findings	MMAT
	undergraduate nursing students' clinical competence.	approach.1031 nursing students included.	77.65% of the variance: perceived learning outcomes, consistency with general clinical performance, quality of assessors, and anxiety/stress impact. • Students' evaluative feedback each semester has been consistently positive. • For many students, the SOAP process provokes anxiety and stress. • While significant improvements have been identified in students' overall performance, the SOAP approach has uncovered a deficit in the learning outcomes of some students.	
Meskell et al. [33] Ireland	To explore electronic objective structured clinical examination (OSCE) delivery and evaluate the benefits of using an electronic OSCE management system.To explore assessors' perceptions of and attitudes to the computer-based package.	A study was conducted using electronic software in the management of a four station OSCE assessment with a cohort of first-year undergraduate nursing students delivered over two consecutive years.The quantitative descriptive survey methodology was used to obtain the views of the assessors on the process and outcome of using the software.203 undergraduate students included.	• The overall outcome of the User Acceptance Test was good, with more than 80% of the examiners having agreed that functionalities did make a lot of sense and that they accepted this online OSCE solution. • Electronic software facilitated the storage and analysis of overall group and individual results, thereby offering considerable time savings. • Submission of electronic forms was allowed only when fully completed thus removing the potential for missing data. • The feedback facility allowed the student to receive timely evaluation on their performance and to benchmark their performance against the class.	50%

Source and country	Objectives	Design	Main findings	MMAT
			• Analysis of assessment results can highlight issues around internal consistency being moderate and examiners variability.	
Nilsson et al. [8] Sweden	To develop and validate a new tool intended for measuring self-reported professional competence among both nursing students prior to graduation and among practicing nurses.	Construction of a new scale and evaluation of its psychometric properties.1086 newly graduated nurse students.	• NPC scale shows satisfactory psychometric properties in a sample of newly graduated nurses. • Tool can be used to evaluate the outcomes of nursing education programs, to assess nurses' competences in relation to the needs in healthcare organizations, to identify self-reported competences, and might be used in tailoring introduction programs for newly employed nurses.	100%
Ossenberg et al. [12] Australia	To advance the assessment properties of a new instrument, the ANSAT, and investigate the acceptability of this instrument for the evaluation of the professional competence of nursing students.	Mixed method approach to collect evidence of validity supporting the instrument.23 clinical assessors included.	• Principal components analysis extracted one factor: professional practice competence. • A comparison of total instrument scores between year levels demonstrated a significant difference in each of the clinical domains ($p = 0.000$), suggesting that the instrument is sensitive to differing levels of performance across different year levels. • The ANSAT demonstrated high internal consistency. • Posttest evaluation completed by assessors demonstrated high usability and acceptability for use in common practice settings. • The results of the statistical analysis strongly support the ANSAT as a valid instrument with	25%

Source and country	Objectives	Design	Main findings	MMAT
			high internal consistency and sensitivity to student progression.	
Ulfvarson and Oxelmark [22] Sweden	To develop of a new criterion-based reference tool to assess nursing knowledge and competence in clinical practice, Assessment of Clinical Education (AClEd)	Development of an instrument using the social constructivist process followed by an assessmentFocus group of 5 students and 80 nurses from clinical settings.	• The tool showed the validity in assessing nursing skills not only in the nursing student's ability to perform a task, but also, most importantly, the quality of nursing care. • The validity of the tool relies on the judgment from the profession.	25%
Walsh et al. [7]Canada	To test the psychometric properties of the Novice Objective Structured Clinical Evaluation Tool.	An instrument-testing design.565 nursing students included.	• The tool was found to have adequate construct validity and reliability. • Its stability should be tested by conducting test-retest analysis. • Equivalency dimensions of reliability should be evaluated by looking at interrater reliability. • This tool shows merit for assessing elements of quality and safety education.	50%

Table 1. Characteristics of studies included in the literature review.

The quality of studies identified was mixed (**Table 1**). Two of twelve studies were judged with a low quality score (25%) with the main reasons for the low quality score being the use of a nonrepresentative sample and uncontrolled testing. Four studies were judged with high quality (75%). Three studies were evaluated as moderate quality (50%), and three studies as very high quality (100%).

The studies identified in **Table 1** were heterogonous that is why they were transformed into qualitative findings using a narrative synthesis [25]. The results were grouped into four assemblages according to the thematic approach: assessment tools, objective structured clinical examination (OSCE), complex assessment approaches, and other approaches.

3.3. Assessment tools

Hsu and Hsieh [21] developed an instrument known as the Competency Inventory of Nursing Students (CINSs) for measuring nursing students' competencies and testing psychometric qualities of baccalaureate nursing students in Taiwan. They used a cross-sectional survey including 599 nursing students. This inventory assesses eight categories that cover ethics and accountability, general clinical skills, lifelong learning, biomedical science, caring, critical thinking, communication, and team working. Ulfvarson and Oxelmark [22] used the social constructivist process to develop a tool for assessing knowledge, and clinical practice contains four domains: nursing, documentation, caring, and skills and manual handling. The tool was tested and found to be valid to measure nursing skills not only of the nursing student's ability to perform a task but also the quality of nursing care. This Assessment of Clinical Education (AClEd) tool evaluated learning outcomes during clinical practice. MMAT score for this study was very low, only 25%. The reliability of the assessment tool was not detected. Nilsson et al. [8] developed a Nurse Professional Competence (NPC) scale for measuring self-reported professional competence that covers eight factors: nursing care, value-based nursing care, medical/technical care, teaching/learning and support, documentation and information technology, legislation in nursing and safety planning, leadership in the development of nursing care, education, and supervision of staff/students. They developed a new scale and evaluated its psychometric properties on a large sample of newly graduated nurse students (n = 1086) from 11 educational institutions in Sweden. This tool can be used to estimate the outcomes of nursing education programs. It can assess nurses' competence in relation to the needs of healthcare organizations, and it can help identify self-reported capabilities and assist in modifying introduction programs for newly employed nurses [8]. Face validity was evaluated by asking students to critically review the item and their understanding of the item within the questionnaire. The data quality was described by mean score, and the construct validity and reliability were described with orthogonal rotation [8]. We recorded the MMAT score for Nilsson et al.'s [8] study very high (100%). Ossenberg et al. [12] based their Australian Nursing Standards Assessment Tool (ANSAT) on the National Competency Standards for the Registered Nurse in Australia, covering professional practice, critical thinking and analysis, provision and coordination of care, and collaborative and therapeutic practice. The validation and acceptability of ANSAT was conducted in a pilot study on 23 clinical assessors, interviews, and with the posttest survey. The recorded MMAT score of study was 25%. More psychometric testing is needed to address current deficits [34]. Iglesias-Parra et al. [30] developed an evaluation system of clinical competencies for the practicum of nursing students based on the Nursing Interventions Classification (NIC). They have prepared a list of 73 NIC interventions that were associated with each of the 26 competencies in nine domains. They took a psychometric validation study in two phases and the cross-sectional study on the population of undergraduate nursing students and clinical tutors. It was found that the competency system, structured on the NIC assessment tool, is a reliable method for assessing and evaluating nursing interventions. Reliability and construct validity were tested by the clinical mentors on 107 students. The survey was conducted with the Delphi technique. The MMAT score was very high (100%). The assessment tool represents a multidimensional approach in formative and combined assessing [30].

3.4. Objective structured clinical examination

Meskell et al. [33] and Walsh et al. [7] both examined OSCE. Meskell et al. [33] evaluated the benefits of using an electronic OSCE assessment system in undergraduate students (n = 203). The electronic software facilitated the storage and analysis of results, thus offering significant time savings. Walsh et al. [7] were focused on the development of a Novice OSCE that included the following competencies: safety, asepsis, knowledge, organization, and caring. An instrument-testing design on a sample of nursing students (n = 565) was used. The MMAT score of both papers was 50%. Some psychometric analysis, reliability, and stability of OSCE tool should be done. OSCE is shown as a formative assessing tool, and it is argued that students should also be assessed in critical thinking and problem-solving skills in addition to clinical skills performance [1, 35].

3.5. Complex assessment approaches

Three studies focused on more complex approaches. Athlin et al. [28] developed a model of a National Clinical Final Examination (NCFE). Their model integrates knowledge from theoretical and practical studies and includes knowledge, skills, capacity of critical thinking, problem-solving, ethical reasoning, independence, and readiness to act. They prepared a two-part examination. This included a written theoretical test with problem-solving characteristics and a bedside test performing nursing care by using observation. Their model was used to assess theoretical and practical knowledge. They found that the model was highly appreciated, and its relevance, usability, and validity were considered as "quite good" for the assessment of nursing students' clinical competence at the final stage of their education. This study recorded a high MMAT score (75%). There is a need to evaluate the model on extensive students' groups because the study was completed using a relatively small sample in theoretical test (n = 73) and a bedside test (n = 68). The model for evaluation of theoretical and practical knowledge used a holistic approach with opportunities for feedback and reflection for students. Imanipour and Jalili [31] developed an assessment system including multiple methods. They used a combination of oral examination and direct observation of a procedural skill. The cognitive knowledge was evaluated by oral exam, and clinical skills were evaluated by direct observation using a global rating scale. The exam includes some generic procedures and two specific procedures. Clinical work sampling was used to evaluate undergraduate bachelor of nursing students' (n = 38) professional behavior. They found that the students and instructors were very satisfied with a comprehensive clinical performance assessment system. Levett-Jones et al. [32] describe the design, implementation, and evaluation of the Structured Observation and Assessment of Practice (SOAP) model used to assess the third-year undergraduate nursing students' (n = 1031) clinical competences. While significant enhancements have been identified in students' overall performance, the SOAP approach has discovered an insufficiency in the learning outcomes of some students.

3.6. Other approaches

Khan et al. [14] evaluated nursing students' perceptions about the effectiveness of utilized teaching and learning strategies of clinical education in improving students' knowledge, skills, and attitudes: demonstration, reflection, and problem-based learning, and concept map. They used both qualitative and quantitative methods in a descriptive cross-sectional study of 74 nursing students to identify nursing students' perceptions about the efficacy of the applied teaching and learning strategies used in clinical education. Problem-based learning and the use of concept maps were perceived to be effective teaching and learning strategies. Hengameh et al. [29] compared the routine evaluation method (a subjective judgment of an instructor about general skills of the student during their clinical course, hence the scoring) with direct observation of procedural skills (DOPS) (clinical activities evaluated based on direct observation using the checklists). They found that applying direct observation of procedural skills (DOPS) significantly enhanced clinical skills and students' scores in clinical procedures.

4. Discussion

The aim of this chapter was to review the literature and critically discuss in relation to identified methods of clinical nursing skills assessment and competencies currently used in nursing higher education. Multidimensional approaches in nursing assessment should be based on a number of differing assessments methods [1]. It should be the combination of knowledge, critical thinking, caring and communication [1, 7, 30], problem-solving, and reflection [36]. Holistic assessment was found to encourage students to be more person-centered [37], rather than purely task-oriented [32]. The literature review identified a wide variety of tools and assessment methods, each with their own advantages and disadvantages. Some were evaluated by nursing students, others by nurses and clinical experts. The studies reviewed were completed in different countries from differing nursing education curriculum and this, along with the range of sample size and approaches used, has proved difficult to make any direct comparison. Nurse educators have a responsibility to ensure that graduates are well prepared for the demands and challenges they will encounter in practice [32]. There is a current imperative to implement a modern and appropriate method of clinical evaluation in nursing education [9, 29]. The current trend requires moving from a generic, technical approach to a more holistic model of clinical assessment, which supports the nurturing and development of competent nursing professionals [34]. The OSCE is a practical test [17, 38] in a simulation area, where the student shows the skills [22] and technical performance [7]. It is also a well-established method to assess clinical skills [33], using a checklist [1] to assess all students with the same set of criteria in order to determine the level of competency achieved in their performance [17, 39]. It provides a level of objectivity in how competency is assessed [32]. The review identified a number of benefits from using OSCE including the achievement of deeper meaningful learning [19], deeper consequential learning [20], and an increase in students' confidence in practice [33]. The OSCE was also identified as a means to facilitate the assessment of psychomotor skills, as well as knowledge and attitudes [20]. As an assessment method, the OSCE helps in the identification of strengths and weaknesses and can focus more on the student getting constructive feedback with or without the consequence of a subsequent examination [40]. In addition to the previous advantages already outlined, Ulfvarson and Oxelmark [22] found that the OSCE can also be used for examining learning outcomes especially those comprising practical skills, such as medical techniques and interpretation of results. It has been recognized as a reliable and valid method to assess clinical skills competency [16, 39–41], and Carraccio and Englander [42] have suggested that the OSCE becomes a key standard for assessing clinical competence. Some criticisms of the OSCE have, however, been identified.

The lack of authenticity due to students not being observed in a real clinical context was identified by Levett-Jones et al. [32], and they further criticized how the OSCE focused on the measurement of technical skills rather than the whole caring situation including the use examination of empathy and interpersonal relationships. The OSCE, however, should be used in conjunction with other evaluation methods [36, 43]. Evaluation methods should be coherent with curriculum and learning out comes. The holistic evaluation methods motivate nursing students' learning, stimulates critical reflective thinking, and make their readiness for professional practice more preferable. Good assessment tools should also be valid and reliable [44].

4.1. Implications for nursing education

Assessment of clinical nursing skills requires collaboration between clinical partners and academia to enhance the clinical experiences of students, the professional development of preceptors or mentors, and the clinical credibility of academics [34]. The findings from the literature review represent a first opportunity to prepare our own assessment tools, according to the cultural and clinical environment, material and economic conditions, national nursing standards, capabilities and purposes of nursing care in Slovenia. There is now an opportunity for all educational institutions with the nursing study programs in the country to prepare assessment tool with cooperation of students, educational experts, and clinical nursing experts.

4.2. Limitations

The findings from the literature review must be considered with respect to the limitations of the studies reviewed and the methods used. Some relevant work may have been omitted due to the inclusion of material only in the English language. The methodological quality of included studies varied from very low [12, 22] to very high [8, 29]. The validity and reliability of the different approaches used were not always discussed, and therefore, our conclusions should be drawn with caution. The MMAT is considered as an efficient tool, although its reliability could be further improved as it appraises only the methodological quality of included studies and not the quality of their reporting [45, 46]. Narrative summary is considered as a more informal approach and can, therefore, be subject to criticism, because of its lack of transparency [27].

5. Conclusion

Despite the heterogeneity of designs and methodology, the findings from the literature review present an overview of current clinical skills assessment tools in practice and in the simulation environment. The assessment of nursing students should include a variety of methods and procedures. It should include the assessment of knowledge, clinical skills, and critical problem-solving in nursing care. There is a need for further research to develop a holistic clinical assessment tool with a reasonable level of validity and reliability, and it must be tested before being applied to the nursing curriculum.

Author details

Nataša Mlinar Reljić*, Mateja Lorber, Dominika Vrbnjak, Brian Sharvin and Maja Strauss

*Address all correspondence to: natasa.mlinar@um.si

Faculty of Health Sciences, University of Maribor, Maribor, Slovenia

References

[1] Cant R, McKenna L, Cooper S. Assessing preregistration nursing students' clinical competence: a systematic review of objective measures. International Journal of Nursing Practice. 2013;**19**(2):162–176. DOI: 10.1111/ijn.12053

[2] Murray E, Gruppen L, Catton P, Hays R, Woolliscroft JO. The accountability of clinical education: its definition and assessment. Medical Education. 2000;**34**(10):871–879. DOI: 10.1046/j.1365-2923.2000.00757.x

[3] McCarthy B, Murphy S. Assessing undergraduate nursing students in clinical practice: do preceptors use assessment strategies?. Nurse Education Today. 2008;**28**(3):301–313. DOI: 10.1016/j.nedt.2007.06.002

[4] Nicol DJ, Macfarlane-Dick D. Formative assessment and self-regulated learning: a model and seven principles of good feedback practice. Studies in Higher Education. 2006;**31** (2):199–218. DOI: 10.1080/03075070600572090

[5] Townsend AH, McLlvenny S, Miller CJ, Dunn EV. The use of an objective structured clinical examination (OSCE) for formative and summative assessment in a general practice clinical attachment and its relationship to final medical school examination performance. Medical Education. 2001;**35**(9):841–846. DOI: 10.1046/j.1365-2923.2001.00957.x

[6] Goodwin LD, Leech NL. The meaning of validity in the new standards for educational and psychological testing: implications for measurement courses. Measurement and Evaluation in Counseling and Development. 2003;**36**(3):181–191.

[7] Walsh M, Bailey PH, Mossey S, Koren I. The novice objective structured clinical evaluation tool: psychometric testing. Journal of Advanced Nursing. 2010;**66**(12):2807–2818. DOI: 10.1111/j.1365-2648.2010.05421.x

[8] Nilsson J, Johansson E, Egmar AC, Florin J, Leksell J, Lepp M, et al. Development and validation of a new tool measuring nurses self-reported professional competence—the Nurse Professional Competence (NPC) scale. Nurse Education Today. 2014;**34**(4):574–580. DOI: 10.1016/j.nedt.2013.07.016

[9] Fotheringham D. Triangulation for the assessment of clinical nursing skills: a review of theory, use and methodology. International Journal of Nursing Studies. 2010;**47**(3):386–391. DOI: 10.1016/j.ijnurstu.2009.09.004

[10] Oermann MH, Yarbrough SS, Saewert KJ, Ard N, Charasika ME. Clinical evaluation and grading practices in schools of nursing: national survey findings part II. Nursing Education Perspectives. 2009;**30**(6):352–357.

[11] Norcini J, Burch V. Workplace-based assessment as an educational tool: AMEE guide no. 31. Medical Teacher. 2007;**29**(9–10):855–871. DOI: 10.1080/01421590701775453

[12] Ossenberg C, Dalton M, Henderson A. Validation of the Australian Nursing Standards Assessment Tool (ANSAT): a pilot study. Nurse Education Today. 2016;**36**:23–30. DOI: 10.1016/j.nedt.2015.07.012

[13] Hartigan I, Murphy S, Flynn AV, Walshe N. Acute nursing episodes which challenge graduate's competence: perceptions of registered nurses. Nurse Education in Practice. 2010;**10**(5):291–297. DOI: 10.1016/j.nepr.2010.01.005

[14] Khan BA, Ali F, Vazir N, Barolia R, Rehan S. Students' perceptions of clinical teaching and learning strategies: a Pakistani perspective. Nurse Education Today. 2012;**32**(1):85–90. DOI: 10.1016/j.nedt.2011.01.016

[15] Kok J, Chabeli MM. Reflective journal writing: how it promotes reflective thinking in clinical nursing education: a students' perspective. Curationis. 2002;**25**(3):35–42.

[16] Yanhua C, Watson R. A review of clinical competence assessment in nursing. Nurse Education Today. 2011;**31**(8):832–836. DOI: 10.1016/j.nedt.2011.05.003

[17] Oranye NO, Ahmad C, Ahmad N, Bakar RA. Assessing nursing clinical skills competence through objective structured clinical examination (OSCE) for open distance learning students in Open University Malaysia. Contemporary Nurse. 2012;**41**(2):233–241. DOI: 10.5172/conu.2012.41.2.233

[18] Alinier G. Nursing students' and lecturers' perspectives of objective structured clinical examination incorporating simulation. Nurse Education Today. 2003;**23**(6):419–426. DOI: 10.1016/S0260-6917(03)00044-3

[19] Barry M, Noonan M, Bradshaw C, Murphy-Tighe S. An exploration of student midwives' experiences of the objective structured clinical examination assessment process. Nurse Education Today. 2012;**32**(6):690–694. DOI: 10.1016/j.nedt.2011.09.007

[20] Baid H. The objective structured clinical examination within intensive care nursing education. Nursing in Critical Care. 2011;**16**(2):99–105. DOI: 10.1111/j.1478-5153.2010.00396.x

[21] Hsu LL, Hsieh SI. Development and psychometric evaluation of the competency inventory for nursing students: a learning outcome perspective. Nurse Education Today. 2013;**33**(5):492–497. DOI: 10.1016/j.nedt.2012.05.028

[22] Ulfvarson J, Oxelmark L. Developing an assessment tool for intended learning outcomes in clinical practice for nursing students. Nurse Education Today. 2012;**32**(6):703–708. DOI: 10.1016/j.nedt.2011.09.010

[23] Nielsen C, Sommer I, Larsen K, Bjørk IT. Model of practical skill performance as an instrument for supervision and formative assessment. Nurse Education in Practice. 2013;**13**(3):176–180. DOI: 10.1016/j.nepr.2012.08.014

[24] Pluye P, Robert E, Cargo M, Bartlett G, O'Cathain A, Griffiths F, et al. Proposal: a Mixed Methods Appraisal Tool for systematic mixed studies reviews [Internet]. 2011. Available from: http://mixedmethodsappraisaltoolpublic.pbworks.com/w/file/fetch/84371689/MMAT 2011 criteria and tutorial 2011-06-29updated2014.08.21.pdf [Accessed: 2016-09-22]

[25] Pluye P, Hong QN. Combining the power of stories and the power of numbers: mixed methods research and mixed studies reviews. Annual Review of Public Health. 2014;**35**:29–45. DOI: 10.1146/annurev-publhealth-032013-182440

[26] Harrison R, Birks Y, Hall J, Bosanquet K, Harden M, Iedema R. The contribution of nurses to incident disclosure: a narrative review. International Journal of Nursing Studies. 2014;**51**(2):334–345. DOI: 10.1016/j.ijnurstu.2013.07.001

[27] Dixon-Woods M, Agarwal S, Jones D, Young B, Sutton A. Synthesising qualitative and quantitative evidence: a review of possible methods. Journal of Health Services Research & Policy. 2005;**10**(1):45–53.

[28] Athlin E, Larsson M, Söderhamn O. A model for a National Clinical Final Examination in the Swedish bachelor programme in nursing. Journal of Nursing Management. 2012;**20** (1):90–101. DOI: 10.1111/j.1365-2834.2011.01278.x

[29] Hengameh H, Afsaneh R, Morteza K, Hosein M, Marjan SM, Abbas E. The effect of applying direct observation of procedural skills (DOPS) on nursing students' clinical skills: a randomized clinical trial. Global Journal of Health Science. 2015;**7**(7):17–21. DOI: 10.5539/gjhs.v7n7p17

[30] Iglesias-Parra MR, García-Guerrero A, García-Mayor S, Kaknani-Uttumchandani S, León-Campos Á, Morales-Asencio JM. Design of a competency evaluation model for clinical nursing practicum, based on standardized language systems: psychometric validation study. Journal of Nursing Scholarship. 2015;**47**(4):371–376. DOI: 10.1111/jnu.12140

[31] Imanipour M, Jalili M. Development of a comprehensive clinical performance assessment system for nursing students: a programmatic approach. Japan Journal of Nursing Science. 2016;**13**(1):46–54. DOI: 10.1111/jjns.12085

[32] Levett-Jones T, Gersbach J, Arthur C, Roche J. Implementing a clinical competency assessment model that promotes critical reflection and ensures nursing graduates' readiness for professional practice. Nurse Education in Practice. 2011;**11**(1):64–69. DOI: 10.1016/j.nepr.2010.07.004

[33] Meskell P, Burke E, Kropmans TJ, Byrne E, Setyonugroho W, Kennedy KM. Back to the future: an online OSCE management information system for nursing OSCEs. Nurse Education Today. 2015;**35**(11):1091–1096. DOI: 10.1016/j.nedt.2015.06.010

[34] Wu XV, Enskär K, Lee CC, Wang W. A systematic review of clinical assessment for undergraduate nursing students. Nurse Education Today. 2015;**35**(2):347–359. DOI: 10.1016/j.nedt.2014.11.016

[35] Cowan DT, Norman I, Coopamah VP. Competence in nursing practice: a controversial concept—a focused review of literature. Nurse Education Today. 2005;**25**(5):355–362. DOI: 10.1016/j.nedt.2005.03.002

[36] Mitchell ML, Henderson A, Groves M, Dalton M, Nulty D. The objective structured clinical examination (OSCE): optimising its value in the undergraduate nursing curriculum. Nurse Education Today. 2009;**29**(4):398–404. DOI: 10.1016/j.nedt.2008.10.007

[37] Laird EA, McCance T, McCormack B, Gribben B. Patients' experiences of in-hospital care when nursing staff were engaged in a practice development programme to promote person-centredness: a narrative analysis study. International Journal of Nursing Studies. 2014;**52**(9):1454–1462. DOI: 10.1016/j.ijnurstu.2015.05.002

[38] Ahuja J. OSCE: a guide for students, part 1. Practice Nurse. 2009;**37**(1):37–39.

[39] Robbins LK, Hoke MM. Using objective structured clinical examinations to meet clinical competence evaluation challenges with distance education students. Perspectives in Psychiatric Care. 2008;**44**(2):81–88. DOI: 10.1111/j.1744-6163.2008.00157.x

[40] McWilliam P, Botwinski C. Developing a successful nursing objective structured clinical examination. Journal of Nursing Education. 2010;**49**(1):36–41. DOI: 10.3928/01484834-20090915-01

[41] Jones A, Pegram A, Fordham-Clarke C. Developing and examining an objective structured clinical examination. Nurse Education Today. 2010;**30**(2):137–141. DOI: 10.1016/j.nedt.2009.06.014

[42] Carraccio C, Englander R. The objective structured clinical examination: a step in the direction of competency-based evaluation. Archives of Pediatrics & Adolescent Medicine. 2000;**154**(17):736–741. DOI: 10.1001/archpedi.154.7.736

[43] van der Vleuten CP, Schuwirth LW, Driessen EW, Dijkstra J, Tigelaar D, Baartman LK, et al. A model for programmatic assessment fit for purpose. Medical Teacher. 2012;**34**(3):205–214. DOI: 10.3109/0142159X.2012.652239

[44] Whiting PF, Rutjes AW, Westwood ME, Mallett S, Deeks JJ, Reitsma JB, et al. QUADAS-2: a revised tool for the quality assessment of diagnostic accuracy studies. Annals of Internal Medicine. 2011;**155**(8):529–536. DOI: 10.7326/0003-4819-155-8-201110180-00009

[45] Souto RQ, Khanassov V, Hong QN, Bush PL, Vedel I, Pluye P. Systematic mixed studies reviews: updating results on the reliability and efficiency of the Mixed Methods Appraisal Tool. International Journal of Nursing Studies. 2015;**52**(1):500–501. DOI: 10.1016/j.ijnurstu.2014.08.010

[46] Vrbnjak D, Denieffe S, O'Gorman C, Pajnkihar M. Barriers to reporting medication errors and near misses among nurses: a systematic review. International Journal of Nursing Studies. 2016;**63**:162–178. DOI: 10.1016/j.ijnurstu.2016.08.019

Impact of Education, Working Conditions, and Interpersonal Relationships on Caregivers' Job Satisfaction

Majda Pajnkihar, Klavdija Čuček Trifkovič,
Barbara Donik, Sabina Fijan, Vida Gönc,
Barbara Kegl, Mateja Lorber, Maja Strauss,
Jadranka Stričević, Sonja Šostar Turk, Gregor Štiglic,
Natalya Nikolaevna Kamynina,
Irina V. Ostrovskaya and Dominika Vrbnjak

Additional information is available at the end of the chapter

http://dx.doi.org/10.5772/67957

Abstract

Aim: To explore relationships between caregivers' education, healthcare working conditions, interpersonal relationships, and caregivers' general job satisfaction.

Background: Caregivers job satisfaction is related to several organizational work environment factors, interpersonal relationships, and personal variables such as education and work experience. Research is needed to understand these variables in different countries due to cultural differences, educational background, and different labor markets.

Design: Cross-sectional multicentre survey.

Methods: Survey data were collected from a convenience sample of 1098 caregivers in five Slovene health care institutions in 2012. Statistical analyzes were undertaken using a descriptive and inferential statistics.

Results: No statistically significant differences were found regarding caregivers' education, average lengths of service, and number of working hours on caregivers' job satisfaction. Job rewards and opportunities predicted higher job satisfaction in nurses with diploma degree. Professional empowerment, supervisor and interpersonal relationships with physicians predicted nursing assistants' higher job satisfaction. Job demands were associated with lower job satisfaction in nursing assistants.

Conclusion: This study contributes to an understanding of the contributing factors of caregivers' general job satisfaction. Results have a great practical value for research, practice, education, and management in the health care system in Slovenia and similar countries.

Keywords: job satisfaction, nursing, working environment, interpersonal relationships, education

1. Introduction

A caring nurse and a conducive working environment influence patients' health outcomes such as patients' satisfaction [1, 2]. Patients' satisfaction can be especially influenced by nurses' job satisfaction [3, 4], which is also related to patients' safety and quality of care [5]. Job satisfaction among nurses has been identified as a key factor in nurses' recruitment and retention, but a comprehensive understanding of nurses' job satisfaction and its related factors remains elusive [6]. It is a critical issue for healthcare organizations in recent years, particularly in nursing, because of potential nurses' shortages, their effect on patients' care, and the associated costs. Rapid changes in healthcare and everyday higher patient expectations and awareness of their rights as well as cross border healthcare treatment have also placed more demands on nurses and this has increased the need for organizations to consider ways to sustain and improve nurses' job satisfaction. To achieve this, they need to understand the factors that affect job satisfaction and dissatisfaction [7]. Hospital leaders need information about factors that underlie nurses' job satisfaction so as to prevent nurses' from leaving their jobs [8] and to improve autonomy, empowerment, and decision-making opportunities in their working environment [9] as well as planning for necessary improvements in practice. More research is required to understand the relative importance of the many identified factors relating to job satisfaction of hospital caregivers [6]. Job satisfaction has an impact on professional work, motivation to achieve results, emphatic relationships with coworkers and patients, and on their personal lives.

2. Background

2.1. Job satisfaction

Job satisfaction is defined as the degree of positive effect toward a job and its main components which is influenced by both, working environment and personal characteristics [10]. General job satisfaction refers to the work environment and the relationship between the employees [11]. Nurses' professional status and their value, autonomy, and professional and personal partner-like relationships within teams and with patients and their families are the most important contributing factors to caregivers' job satisfaction [12]. Interpersonal relationships are especially important and are stimulated in the workplace. Results by

Tzeng and Ketefian [3] showed that nurses' general job satisfaction, general feelings of happiness when they are doing their jobs, and their job satisfaction are significantly correlated with inpatient satisfaction, such as explanation of care, art of care, pain management, and arrangement for home care and follow up. Nurses' job dissatisfaction could be reflected in nurses' attitudes and behaviors, adversely affecting nurse-patient interactions and patients' perceptions of those interactions [4]. Interactions between coworkers could also be affected. Nurses' job dissatisfaction is related with the intent to leave [13] and a key factor in nurse' turnover [6]. Job satisfaction is related to a number of organizational, professional, and personal variables [6]. It can be influenced by different working conditions and interpersonal relationships. In addition, nurses' educational background should be considered as an important factor in understanding nurses' job satisfaction [6, 14]. It seems that nurses with tertiary education are less satisfied with their jobs than those who had not received tertiary education [6]. In Slovenia, there are 72% (n = 12,387) of caregivers with 4-year secondary vocational education (nursing assistants) and 28% (n = 4871) of caregivers with higher or tertiary education in nursing (nurses with diploma degree) [15]. Different issues have greater significance in different countries due to the social context of the different labor markets [6].

2.2. Working conditions and interpersonal relationships

Adequate staffing and resources [16–20], workload and working hours [21], nursing management [8, 17, 22–25], autonomy and decision-making [17, 25–28], status, recognition, job and task requirements, opportunity for advancement [25], and also employee engagement and commitment [29] are frequently reported working conditions that have an impact on nurses' job satisfaction. Listed conditions represent professional characteristics that are strongly associated with intra- and interprofessional relationships that exist in the workplace. For nurses, job satisfaction is the most important nurse physician relationships [4] following interpersonal relationships, such as human relationships with coworkers, feeling of togetherness, interaction and communication, teamwork, and peer support [17, 23].

3. The study

3.1. Aim

The main aim of this study was to explore relationships between caregivers' education, healthcare working conditions, interpersonal relationships, and caregivers' general job satisfaction. We proposed the following research question: "What is the impact of education, working conditions, and interpersonal relationships on caregivers' general job satisfaction."

3.2. Design

The study used a cross-sectional multicentre survey conducted among nursing assistants and nurses with diploma degree.

3.3. Setting and participants

We collected data from five different health care institutions in Slovenia including a range of hospital types from large university clinical centers to small general hospitals and different units. Convenience sampling was used. Questionnaires were distributed to 1098 caregivers representing 29.84% of 3680 caregivers working in the included five healthcare institutions and 11.68% of 9404 caregivers in all Slovenian hospitals. A total of 613 questionnaires were returned, giving a response rate of 55.83%.

3.4. Data collection

Data collection took place in August 2012. The researchers handed out questionnaires to caregivers in different units of the five health care institutions, including nursing assistants (4-years of secondary vocational education) and nurses with a diploma degree (3-years of higher education in nursing). Return of completed questionnaires was considered as a consent for participation. The completed questionnaires for nurses were returned in a sealed box clearly identifiable in the ward. This box was regularly emptied by researchers.

3.5. Ethical considerations

Approval was obtained from all five healthcare institutions that provided a written permission for research. Caregivers were informed about the study aims prior to administration of the questionnaires.

3.6. Instruments

The survey was adapted from previous research in the United States [29, 30]. Caregivers' education was measured at the individual level. We also used an average length of service on each of study units and caregivers working hours per week on a unit. The work environment was measured using a questionnaire Supports for Individual and Team Performance [29, 30]. The questionnaire contains 54 items related to support for individual and team performance and uses a 1-to-5 Likert scale with the following levels: 1—"Never," 2—"Rarely," 3—"Some of the time," 4—"Most of the time," and 5—"All of the time." Respondents circled the number best corresponding their belief about the statement, where 1 represents never and 5 represents all the time. Items are grouped into eight subscales: hospital decision-making (5-items), staffing and resources (5-items), job demands (3-items), professional empowerment (11-items), job rewards and opportunities (8-items), supervisory relationships (12-items), delivering patient-centered care (4-items), and communication about patients (6-items). Interpersonal relationships were measured using the Team Effectiveness questionnaire. Interpersonal relationships with physicians (10-items), nurses with a diploma degree (10-items), and nursing assistants (10-items) were assessed. The questionnaire uses a 1-to-5 Likert scale with the same levels as in the support for individual team performance questionnaire. Nurses satisfaction was measured using a single question "Overall, how satisfied are you with your job?" It was represented by a Likert scale consisting of the following four options: "Very satisfied", "Somewhat satisfied", "Somewhat dissatisfied" and "Very dissatisfied".

3.7. Validity and reliability

The work environment was measured using a survey item previously used in the United States to research the support for individual and team performance. The original survey was based on the Revised Nursing Work Index, developed by Aiken and Patrician (2000), the Picker Hospital Employee Survey, developed by The Picker Institute (2006), and tools from workplace settings in industries outside of health care, particularly those related to high-performance work systems and teams developed by Weinberg and her team. Unlike the Nursing Work Index, the tool went beyond nursing and examined structural supports for healthcare work for multiple providers. Combined Cronbach's alpha of the original survey was 0.81 [30]. The Slovene version was translated by a professional translator using a standardized translation. Content validity, acceptability, and feasibility of the survey were assured through a nursing group research discussion, including a group of six experienced nursing researchers. Questions regarding caregivers' education and caregivers working hours per week on a unit were adapted to Slovene working conditions. Combined Cronbach's alpha of the Supports for Individual and Team Performance survey was 0.89 and 0.94 for the Team Effectiveness Questionnaire.

3.8. Data analysis

Data were analyzed using R, version 3.0.3 (http://cran.org). Descriptive statistics were used to describe caregivers' education, average lengths of service on each of the study units and caregivers working hours per week on a unit. Exploratory analysis was conducted by visualization of the job satisfaction mean value with corresponding 95% confidence intervals for compared groups based on the education, length of service, and weekly working hours.

Additionally, we examined how nurse job satisfaction relates to level of education, eight measures of individual or team performance (ITP), and interpersonal relations (IR). The eight measures of ITP consisted of the following subscales: hospital decision-making, staffing and resources, job demands, professional empowerment, job rewards and opportunities, your supervisor, delivering patient centered care, and communication about patients. Three measures of interpersonal relationships (IR) consisted of the following units: interpersonal relationships with physicians, interpersonal relationships with nursing assistants, and interpersonal relationships with nurses with diploma degree. Level of education was defined as high (nurses with diploma degree) and low (nursing assistants), since most of the caregivers in our study belonged to these two groups.

First, we compared mean values with corresponding confidence intervals for all measures of ITP and IR in both groups based on education. Mean values of both groups were compared using the nonparametric Mann-Whitney U-test for two independent samples. Benjamini and Hochberg [31] procedure was used to control for the false discovery rate due to multiple testing.

Finally, we built two regression models to explore relations between job satisfaction and 11 numeric predictors in two groups of different education level. The output variable of ordinal logistic regression (OLR) models was represented by job satisfaction level and was based on a question "Overall, how satisfied are you with your job?" It was represented by four ordinal values, including 1—"Very satisfied," 2—"Somewhat satisfied," 3—"Somewhat dissatisfied," and 4—"Very dissatisfied." Eleven numeric predictors with average ITP and IR subscale scores for each individual were used as predictors. Statistical significance was set at $P < 0.05$.

Participants with missing values were excluded from the model building process. Therefore, the OLR models were built using 293 for low and 246 samples for high education level.

4. Results

Most caregivers belonged to the group of nursing assistants ($n = 327$, 53.3%) and nurses with a diploma degree ($n = 266$, 43.3%). Thirteen (2.3%) respondents had the other educational background and were excluded from further analysis. Detailed sample demographic characteristics are presented in **Table 1**.

Demographic characteristics	**Responses**
Education	
Nursing assistants, *n* (%)	327 (53.3%)
Nurses with diploma degree, *n* (%)	266 (43.3%)
Other	13 (2.3%)
Missing	7 (1.1%)
Average lengths of service on selected unit, *n* (%)	
Less than one year	53 (8.6%)
1–2 years	68 (11.1%)
3–4 years	67 (10.9%)
More than four years	418 (68.2%)
Missing	7 (1.1%)
Weekly working hours, *n* (%)	
Under 40 hours per week	78 (12.7%)
40 hours per week	187 (30.5%)
Over 40 hours per week	337 (55%)
Missing	7 (1.1%)
Gender, *n* (%)	
Female	526 (85.8%)
Male	80 (13.1%)
Missing	7 (1.1%)

Table 1. Demographic characteristics.

In an additional analysis of relations between the job satisfaction, working conditions, and interpersonal relationships, we analyzed the relation between the job satisfaction and length of service (**Figure 1**). Although we could not find any statistically significant differences between the observed groups for any length of service, one can notice the trend in the gap between the two groups that is increasing with the length of service.

Figure 2 also explores the differences in job satisfaction between the two observed groups and focuses on the weekly working hours expressed in three groups—participants working less, exactly, or more than 40 hours per week. One can observe a decrease in the job satisfaction difference between the observed groups with the increased weekly working hours. None of the differences are statistically significant.

Table 2 presents a summary of individual or team performance and interpersonal relationship predictors for nursing assistants and nurses with a diploma degree. The lowest mean value in the group of nursing assistants was found in ITP decision making ($M = 1.43$, 95% CI 1.34–1.52) and the lowest mean value in the group of nurses with a diploma degree for ITP job rewards and opportunities ($M = 1.69$, 95% CI 1.61–1.78). The highest mean value in the group of nursing assistants was found in IR with nursing assistants ($M = 4.38$, 95% CI 4.32–4.44) and in the group of nurses with a diploma degree for IR with Nurses with Diploma Degree ($M = 4.22$, 95% 4.16–4.28). Statistically significant differences in mean values of both groups were found in ITP Decision Making, IR with Nursing Assistants, and IR with Nurses with a Diploma Degree ($P < 0.001$).

Table 3 represents the results of OLR and corresponding significance values within a group of Nursing Assistants. It should be noted that 1—"Very satisfied" translates to the highest level of job satisfaction, meaning that negative regression coefficients contribute to higher satisfaction. Within the group of Nursing Assistants, Job Demands is a predictor with a positive coefficient that results in 0.632 units' lower job satisfaction for each unit of increase in ITP

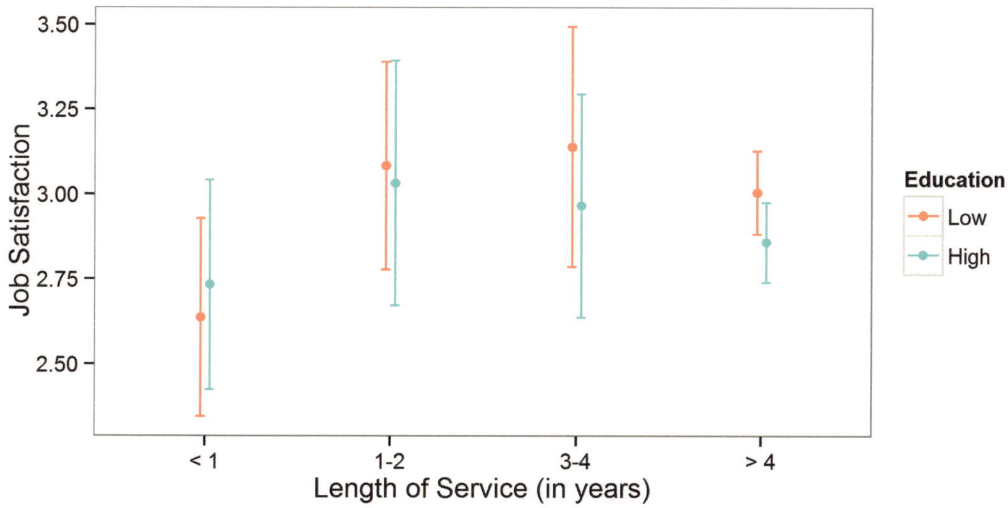

Figure 1. Comparison of job satisfaction for two groups of participants based on their education for different lengths of service.

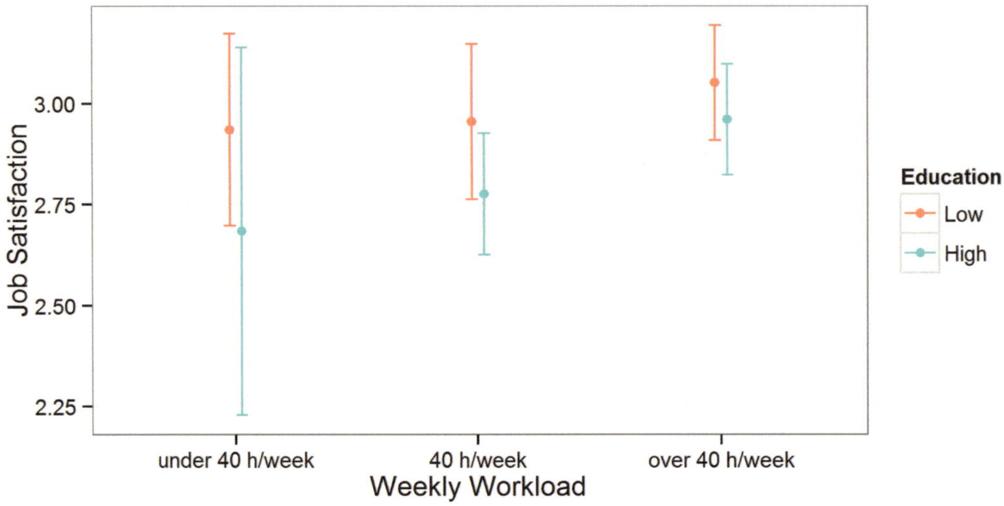

Figure 2. Comparison of job satisfaction for two groups of participants based on their education for different weekly working hours.

Predictor	Nursing assistants		RNs with diploma		Mann-Whitney *P* value
	Mean	95 % CI	Mean	95% CI	
ITP hospital decision-making	1.43	1.34–1.52	1.72	1.61–1.82	**<0.001**
ITP staffing and resources	2.46	2.38–2.54	2.46	2.39–2.54	1.000
ITP job demands	2.80	2.74–2.87	2.77	2.70–2.84	0.409
ITP professional empowerment	2.97	2.93–3.02	3.02	2.97–3.06	0.305
ITP job rewards and opportunities	1.59	1.51–1.67	1.69	1.61–1.78	0.108
ITP supervisor	2.23	2.17–2.28	2.30	2.24–2.36	0.108
ITP delivering patient-centered care	3.17	3.10–3.24	3.16	3.09–3.23	0.958
ITP communication about patients	2.55	2.46–2.63	2.58	2.50–2.65	0.694
IR with physicians	3.70	3.63–3.77	3.74	3.67–3.81	0.430
IR with nursing assistants	4.38	4.32–4.44	4.12	4.04–4.19	**<0.001**
IR with nurses with diploma degree	3.97	3.90–4.05	4.22	4.16–4.28	**<0.001**

All p-values below 0.05 are mentioned in bold.

Table 2. Summary of individual or team performance and interpersonal relationship predictors for two groups of participants based on education level ($n = 539$).

Job Demands in the log odds scale. Two predictors, Professional Empowerment and Your Supervisor in the measure of an individual or team performance are predictors related to higher job satisfaction. Professional empowerment is a predictor with a negative coefficient −0.872 that results in higher job satisfaction ($P = 0.016$). The supervisor is a predictor with a negative coefficient −0.750 that contributes to higher job satisfaction ($P = 0.011$). In interpersonal relationships measure, only IR with Physicians is a predictor with a negative coefficient

Predictor	Value	Std. error	t value	P value
ITP hospital decision making	0.299	0.183	1.636	0.102
ITP staffing and resources	0.036	0.247	0.150	0.881
ITP job demands	0.632	0.249	2.539	**0.011**
ITP professional empowerment	−0.872	0.363	−2.402	**0.016**
ITP job rewards and opportunities	−0.398	0.224	−1.775	0.076
ITP supervisor	−0.750	0.293	−2.556	**0.011**
ITP delivering patient centered care	−0.052	0.235	−0.223	0.824
ITP communication about patients	0.073	0.207	0.354	0.724
IR with physicians	−0.848	0.259	−3.281	**0.001**
IR with nursing assistants	0.008	0.279	0.027	0.978
IR with nurses with diploma degree	−0.193	0.253	−0.764	0.445

ITP, individual or team performance; IR, interpersonal relations.
All p-values below 0.05 are mentioned in bold.

Table 3. Ordinal logistic regression results for prediction of the job satisfaction level within a group of nursing assistants ($n = 293$).

−0.848 that significantly contributes to higher job satisfaction ($P = 0.001$). All other predictors were not statistically significant for job satisfaction within a group of Nursing Assistants.

Table 4 represents the results of OLR and corresponding significance values within a group of Nurses with Diploma degree. In the group of Nurses with Diploma Degree, only Job Rewards and Opportunities was a significant predictor of job satisfaction, a predictor with a negative coefficient −0.631 that contributed higher job satisfaction ($P = 0.017$).

Predictor	Value	Std. error	t value	P value
ITP hospital decision making	0.005	0.194	0.024	0.981
ITP staffing and resources	−0.011	0.297	−0.036	0.972
ITP job demands	0.395	0.272	1.451	0.147
ITP professional empowerment	0.076	0.371	0.205	0.838
ITP job rewards and opportunities	−0.631	0.264	−2.386	**0.017**
ITP supervisor	−0.615	0.329	−1.872	0.061
ITP delivering patient centered care	0.126	0.261	0.482	0.630
ITP communication about patients	−0.277	0.279	−0.993	0.321
IR with physicians	−0.495	0.277	−1.791	0.073
IR with nursing assistants	−0.137	0.287	−0.4732	0.636
IR with nurses with diploma degree	−0.438	0.356	−1.230	0.219

All p-values below 0.05 are mentioned in bold.

Table 4. Ordinal logistic regression results for prediction of the job satisfaction level within a group of nurses with diploma degree ($n = 246$).

5. Discussion

The aim of our study was to explore the relationships between caregiver education, healthcare working conditions, interpersonal relationships, and caregivers' general job satisfaction.

No statistically significant differences were found regarding caregiver education, lengths of service, and number of working hours on their job satisfaction, which is in contrast to other studies. Lu et al. [6], for example, found that hours of work are a significant predictor of job satisfaction. One of the possible reasons for our results is a small sample size (only 19 nurses with a diploma degree in category working less than 40 hours per week). Additional research using a bigger sample size is needed to confirm this trend. Nonetheless, we can observe a trend between increased weekly working hours and increased job satisfaction. One possible explanation is that caregivers, although facing increased workload, have high job control or high job social support that enhances intrinsic work motivation [32]. Increased weekly working hours could be related also to pay increases, especially if caregivers are working at weekends or night shifts.

Examining the working environment, we found statistical differences within two researched groups of caregivers, nursing assistants, and nurses with diploma degree. In the group of nursing assistants, job demands resulted in lower job satisfaction. Research results showed that they have to work very fast and very hard most of the time. Job demands were found to be a significant factor for caregivers' lower job satisfaction also in Bégat et al. [33], Seo et al. [34], Chu et al. [35], Demerouti et al. [36]. Current nursing work environments are characterized by heavy workloads that contribute to stress among caregivers [37]. That is also true for Slovenian healthcare system, where caregivers are burdened with heavy workloads and are underpaid. We also have a higher proportion of nursing assistants when compared to nurses with diploma degree. So nursing assistants are sometimes responsible also for nursing interventions for which they do not have formally obtained knowledge and competences. This can happen especially in situations of increased workload at wards (i.e., increased number of hospitalization, sick leave). It is, therefore, especially important to establish congruence between nurses' workload and their rewards [36] and job demands.

Regarding the work environment, there were more significant predictors that positively affected job satisfaction in nursing assistants than in nurses with diploma degree. Professional empowerment and supervisor were a significant predictor of nursing assistants' job satisfaction, whereas job rewards and opportunities was the only predictor of higher job satisfaction in nurses with diploma degree. This is not so surprising because nursing assistants need to receive more assistance and resources to enhance their job satisfaction [38]. Our research results showed that nursing assistants estimate the work they do as important and they use their knowledge; however, they need more resources and support.

Professional empowerment is important for job satisfaction, because an employee can be satisfied with the basic content of the job, but may be frustrated if it does not allow one to grow or move into roles in other areas of the organization [39]. Highly educated nurses may have more work opportunities than those with lower levels of education [40], while nursing assistants have less control over their work and less autonomy. That is why they need more opportunities for continuing education [12]. Additionally, nursing assistants wish to improve professional empowerment, thereby creating a positive working environment [12]. In Slovenian hospitals, we have also a lack of a comprehensive career development system [41]. Caregivers in our research claim that they never or rarely have opportunity to get a better job in their respective institution.

Nurse managers have a strong role in promoting nurses' job satisfaction [16, 17, 42]. Attention should be paid especially to strengthen nurses' interpersonal relationships and facilitate nurses' capacity to deliver high-quality patient care [17]. Aiken et al. [13] researched nursing job satisfaction in five different countries with different health care systems and found that fewer than half of the nurses reported that management in their hospitals is responsive to their concerns, provides opportunities for nurses to participate in decision-making, and acknowledges nurses' contributions to patient care. Our research results showed that respect, trust, recognition, support in further education and training and inclusion in decision-making are important factors that should be addressed by nursing administrators in practice.

Our results underline the importance of reward in relation to job satisfaction, as found in different studies [42, 43]. In the group of nurses with diploma degree, only job rewards and opportunities were found to be a significant predictor of higher job satisfaction. Nurses with a diploma degree in Slovenia have much greater autonomy, control over work, better salary, and professional status and are also more empowered when compared to nursing assistants. However, a trend of labor migration can be seen in Slovenia; caregivers search jobs in other western countries, where salaries, working conditions, and career development opportunities are better.

In relation to examining interpersonal relationships, only interpersonal relationships with physicians was a predictor of higher job satisfaction, but again only in nursing assistants group. Nurses' job performance in hospitals is dependent upon their relationships with physicians [44], so nurse-physician collaboration was found to be a major predictor of job satisfaction [45]. This predictor was not significant in nurses with diploma degree. One of the possible reasons of this result is, as already previously stated, lack of autonomy and control over the work in group of nursing assistants. Another possible reason is our legislation that states that physicians are those who are responsible for the complex process of healing and treatment. Physicians and nurses also tend to work together or consult each other at times, whereas nursing assistants tend to have more a hierarchical, subservient relationship with physicians and nurses [46]. Differences between intraprofessional and interprofessional communication is expected because of cultural differences between caregivers and physicians [47], which was also shown by our research results. Caregivers assessed intraprofessional relationships better then interprofessional relationships with physicians. In our healthcare system, hierarchical relationships in healthcare teams are firmly rooted. There should be more emphasis on interdisciplinary and multidisciplinary collaboration. Nurses should be aware of their role of being "connective" [12].

Other research shows that not only nurse-physician relationships but also peer relationships are important contributing factors of nurses' job satisfaction [10, 48]. Utriainen and Kyngäs [17] found that interpersonal relationships such as human relationships with coworkers, feeling of togetherness, interaction and communication, team work, social climate and ethicality, and peer support are important in hospital nurses' satisfaction, which contrasts with of our findings. Interpersonal relationships with peers were not found as a significant predictor of job satisfaction. Nursing assistants and nurses were very satisfied with their interpersonal relationships, mean values for interpersonal relationships with nursing assistants, and interpersonal relationships with nurses with diploma degree were higher in both groups when compared to other predictors and ranged from 3.97 (95% CI 3.90–4.05) to 4.38 (95% CI 4.32–4.44). However, as is evident in **Table 2**, both nursing assistants and nurses with a diploma degree rated communication with their own peers better than communication with group of caregivers with different level of education, and the differences were statistically significant. Hierarchy is present not only within healthcare teams but also in nursing teams. It is also known that nurses usually possess the conceptual knowledge of the meaning of communication and collaboration, but struggle with this in the practice setting [49]. A sense of belonging, being one of them, appreciated, loved, able to rely on coworkers make us feel safe in our workplace so relationships and communication in nursing teams need to be addressed in practice. It is the essence of nursing that professionals are aware of human and equal interpersonal relationship based on trust and respect [12].

The important element that nursing is entitled to and which will help it to gain autonomy and social acknowledgment is academic education. Nursing has achieved a lot through formal education, but it is still in a dependent position relative to other professions, especially to medicine [12].

Nurses' job satisfaction is especially important in the current context of nurse shortages [13], so the results of this study can contribute to the understanding of such a complex phenomenon and will help managers to plan effective interventions. Also in our country, healthcare system is faced with a lack of caregivers because of the economic crisis.

5.1. Limitations

The main limitation of this study is the study design. We have presented a cross-sectional study that cannot positively and accurately confirm the established causalities. Further longitudinal studies are required to confirm our results. Second, convenience sampling of the caregivers was used, so results cannot be generalized.

5.2. Implications for policy/practice/research/education

Results of this study have a great practical value and utility for managers when preparing strategies and selecting a sound nursing theory to support intraprofessional and interprofessional relationships and to assure overall satisfaction of caregivers in countries with similar health care service. Additional research using a larger sample size is needed to confirm trends of increased weekly working hours and increased job satisfaction. Greater emphasis should be placed on lifelong education and training in intraprofessional and interprofessional communication and collaboration. Empowerment, improvement of career development opportunities, and enhancement of professional growth are required by nursing assistants.

6. Conclusion

This study has provided a depiction of the relationships between caregiver education, healthcare working conditions, interpersonal relationships, and caregivers' general job satisfaction. Two factors of working environment, professional empowerment and supervisor, and one factor of interpersonal relationships, interpersonal relationships with physicians were found to be positively affect nursing assistants' job satisfaction. One factor, job demands, was found to negatively affect nursing assistant's job satisfaction. Job satisfaction of nurses with diploma degree was found to be positively affected only by job rewards and opportunities.

The results of this study serve as a good foundation for future studies of these multifactorial and complex phenomena in the healthcare setting. Additional research is needed to confirm and explore trends of increased weekly working hours and increased job satisfaction using not only quantitative approach but also qualitative or mixed methods research.

Results have implication for caregivers' education and training in nursing practice. Greater emphasis on education and training in intraprofessional and interprofessional communication and collaboration should be placed in curricula. Empowerment of nursing assistants, improvement of their career development opportunities, and enhancement of their professional growth is needed. Results have, therefore, a great practical value also for managers in the healthcare system in Slovenia and similar countries. Furthermore, significant strategies should be prepared to assure overall satisfaction of caregivers. Increasing the number of nurses with higher education degree is one of the first steps in ensuring the safety and making progress in the quality, safety, and efficiency of healthcare delivery.

Acknowledgements

This study was partially funded by the Slovenian Research Agency. The study was undertaken as a part of a bilateral research project called Safety and Caring for Patients in a Clinical Environment in Correlation with Education of Nurses between University of Maribor, Faculty of Health Sciences, and I.M. Sechenov First Moscow State Medical University of the Ministry of Health and Social Development. We thank the researchers Y. Brazhnikov, E. Efremova, and Igor S. Lunkov.

Author details

Majda Pajnkihar[1*], Klavdija Čuček Trifkovič[1], Barbara Donik[1], Sabina Fijan[1], Vida Gönc[1], Barbara Kegl[1], Mateja Lorber[1], Maja Strauss[1], Jadranka Stričević[1], Sonja Šostar Turk[1,2], Gregor Štiglic[1,3], Natalya Nikolaevna Kamynina[4], Irina V. Ostrovskaya[4] and Dominika Vrbnjak[1]

*Address all correspondence to: majda.pajnkihar@um.si

1 University of Maribor, Faculty of Health Sciences, Maribor, Slovenia

2 University of Maribor, Faculty of Mechanical Engineering, Maribor, Slovenia

3 University of Maribor, Faculty of Electrical Engineering and Computer Science, Maribor, Slovenia

4 I.M. Sechenov First Moscow State Medical University of the Ministry, Faculty of Higher Nursing Training, Psychology and Social Work of Health and Social Development, Moscow, Russian Federation

References

[1] Cossette S, Cote JK, Pepin J, Ricard N, D'Aoust LX. A dimensional structure of nurse-patient interactions from a caring perspective: refinement of the Caring Nurse-Patient Interaction Scale (CNPI—Short Scale). Journal of Advanced Nursing 2006;55(2):198–214.

[2] Finfgeld-Connett D. Meta-synthesis of caring in nursing. Journal of Clinical Nursing 2008;17(2):196–204.

[3] Tzeng HM, Ketefian S. The relationship between nurses' job satisfaction and inpatient satisfaction: an exploratory study in a Taiwan teaching hospital. Journal of Nursing Care Quality 2002;16(2):39–49.

[4] Larrabee JH, Ostrow CL, Withrow ML, Janney MA, Hobbs GR, Jr., Burant C. Predictors of patient satisfaction with inpatient hospital nursing care. Research in Nursing & Health 2004;27(4):254–68.

[5] Atefi N, Abdullah KL, Wong LP, Mazlom R. Factors influencing registered nurses perception of their overall job satisfaction: a qualitative study. International Nursing Review 2014;61(3):352–60.

[6] Lu H, Barriball KL, Zhang X, While AE. Job satisfaction among hospital nurses revisited: a systematic review. International Journal of Nursing Studies 2012;49(8):1017–38.

[7] Maqbali MA. Factors that influence nurses' job satisfaction: a literature review. Nursing Management (Harrow, London, England: 1994) 2015;22(2):30–7.

[8] Larrabee JH, Janney MA, Ostrow CL, Withrow ML, Hobbs GR, Jr., Burant C. Predicting registered nurse job satisfaction and intent to leave. The Journal of Nursing Administration 2003;33(5):271–83.

[9] Erenstein CF, McCaffrey R. How healthcare work environments influence nurse retention. Holistic Nursing Practice 2007;21(6):303–7.

[10] Adams A, Bond S. Hospital nurses' job satisfaction, individual and organizational characteristics. Journal of Advanced Nursing 2000;32(3):536–43.

[11] Yang J, Liu Y, Chen Y, Pan X. The effect of structural empowerment and organizational commitment on Chinese nurses' job satisfaction. Applied Nursing Research: ANR 2014;27(3):186–91.

[12] Pajnkihar M. Theory development for nursing in Slovenia [PhD thesis] 2003 Manchester: University of Manchester, Faculty of Medicine, Dentistry, Nursing and Pharmacy.

[13] Aiken LH, Clarke SP, Sloane DM, Sochalski JA, Busse R, Clarke H, et al. Nurses' reports on hospital care in five countries. Health Affairs (Millwood) 2001;20(3):43–53.

[14] Cicolini G, Comparcini D, Simonetti V. Workplace empowerment and nurses' job satisfaction: a systematic literature review. Journal of Nursing Management 2014;22(7):855–71.

[15] National Institute of Public Health of the Republic of Slovenia. Izvajalci zdravstvene dejavnosti/Health care resources 2014 [Available from: https://podatki.nijz.si/pxweb/sl/NIJZ%20podatkovni%20portal/NIJZ%20podatkovni%20portal__6%20Zdravstvene%20storitve%20in%20sistem%20zdravstvenega%20varstva__6d%20Izvajalci%20zdravstvene%20dejavnosti/BPI_TB02.px/table/tableViewLayout2/?rxid=feb078b4-3bb6-405b-bfe2-ceba0f2ce56d.

[16] Aiken LH, Clarke SP, Sloane DM. Hospital staffing, organization, and quality of care: cross-national findings. International Journal for Quality in Health Care: Journal of the International Society for Quality in Health Care/ISQua 2002;14(1):5–13.

[17] Utriainen K, Kyngäs H. Hospital nurses' job satisfaction: a literature review. Journal of Nursing Management 2009;17(8):1002–10.

[18] Tervo-Heikkinen T, Kvist T, Partanen P, Vehvilainen-Julkunen K, Aalto P. Patient satisfaction as a positive nursing outcome. Journal of Nursing Care Quality 2008;23(1):58–65.

[19] Bruyneel L, Li B, Ausserhofer D, Lesaffre E, Dumitrescu I, Smith HL, et al. Organization of hospital nursing, provision of nursing care, and patient experiences with care in Europe. Medical Care Research and Review: MCRR 2015;72(6):643–64.

[20] Wolf ZR, Colahan M, Costello A. Relationship between nurse caring and patient satisfaction. Medsurg Nursing: Official Journal of the Academy of Medical-Surgical Nurses 1998;7(2):99–105.

[21] Griffiths P, Dall'Ora C, Simon M, Ball J, Lindqvist R, Rafferty AM, et al. Nurses' shift length and overtime working in 12 European countries: the association with perceived quality of care and patient safety. Medical Care 2014;52(11):975–81.

[22] Upenieks VV. Assessing differences in job satisfaction of nurses in magnet and nonmagnet hospitals. The Journal of Nursing Administration 2002;32(11):564–76.

[23] Cummings GG, Olson K, Hayduk L, Bakker D, Fitch M, Green E, et al. The relationship between nursing leadership and nurses' job satisfaction in Canadian oncology work environments. Journal of Nursing Management 2008;16(5):508–18.

[24] Cummings GG, MacGregor T, Davey M, Lee H, Wong CA, Lo E, et al. Leadership styles and outcome patterns for the nursing workforce and work environment: a systematic review. International Journal of Nursing Studies 2010;47(3):363–85.

[25] Sengin KK. Work-related attributes of RN job satisfaction in acute care hospitals. The Journal of Nursing Administration 2003;33(6):317–20.

[26] Iliopoulou KK, While AE. Professional autonomy and job satisfaction: survey of critical care nurses in mainland Greece. Journal of Advanced Nursing 2010;66(11):2520–31.

[27] Bjork IT, Samdal GB, Hansen BS, Torstad S, Hamilton GA. Job satisfaction in a Norwegian population of nurses: a questionnaire survey. International Journal of Nursing Studies 2007;44(5):747–57.

[28] Roberts-Turner R, Hinds PS, Nelson J, Pryor J, Robinson NC, Wang J. Effects of leadership characteristics on pediatric registered nurses' job satisfaction. Pediatric Nursing 2014;40(5):236–41, 56.

[29] Weinberg DB, Avgar AC, Sugrue NM, Cooney-Miner D. The importance of a high-performance work environment in hospitals. Health Services Research 2013;48(1):319–32.

[30] Weinberg DB, Cooney-Miner D, Perloff JN. Analyzing the relationship between nursing education and patient outcomes. Journal of Nursing Regulation 2012;3(2):1–4.

[31] Benjamini Y, Hochberg Y. Controlling the false discovery rate: a practical and powerful approach to multiple testing. Journal of the Royal Statistical Society Series B (Methodological) 1995:289–300.

[32] Van Yperen NW, Hagedoorn M. Do high job demands increase intrinsic motivation or fatigue or both? The role of job control and job social support. Academy of Management Journal 2003;46(3):339–48.

[33] Bégat I, Ellefsen B, Severinsson E. Nurses' satisfaction with their work environment and the outcomes of clinical nursing supervision on nurses' experiences of well-being—a Norwegian study. Journal of Nursing Management 2005;13(3):221–30.

[34] Seo Y, Ko J, Price JL. The determinants of job satisfaction among hospital nurses: a model estimation in Korea. International Journal of Nursing Studies 2004;41(4):437–46.

[35] Chu CI, Hsu HM, Price JL, Lee JY. Job satisfaction of hospital nurses: an empirical test of a causal model in Taiwan. International Nursing Review 2003;50(3):176–82.

[36] Demerouti E, Bakker AB, Nachreiner F, Schaufeli WB. A model of burnout and life satisfaction amongst nurses. Journal of Advanced Nursing 2000;32(2):454–64.

[37] Spence Laschinger HK, Wilk P, Cho J, Greco P. Empowerment, engagement and perceived effectiveness in nursing work environments: does experience matter? Journal of Nursing Management 2009;17(5):636–46.

[38] Kuo HT, Yin TJ, Li IC. Relationship between organizational empowerment and job satisfaction perceived by nursing assistants at long-term care facilities. Journal of Clinical Nursing 2008;17(22):3059–66.

[39] Lautizi M, Laschinger HK, Ravazzolo S. Workplace empowerment, job satisfaction and job stress among Italian mental health nurses: an exploratory study. Journal of Nursing Management 2009;17(4):446–52.

[40] Yin JC, Yang KP. Nursing turnover in Taiwan: a meta-analysis of related factors. International Journal of Nursing Studies 2002;39(6):573–81.

[41] Skela Savič B, Robida A. Usposobljenost srednjega managementa na področju dela z ljudmi v slovenskih bolnišnicah = Capacity of middle management for working with people in Slovenian hospital. In: Skela Savič B, Hvalič Touzery S, Skinder Savić K, Zurc J, Avberšek-Lužnik I, Bregar B, et al., editors. Zbornik predavanj z recenzijo = Proceedings

http://dx.doi.org/10.5772/67957

of lectures with peer review; 5 mednarodna znanstvena konferenca Kakovostna zdravstvena obravnava skozi izobraževanje, raziskovanje in multiprofesionalno povezovanje – prispevek k zdravju posameznika in družbe, 7–8 junij 2012 = 5th International Scientific Conference Quality Health Care Treatment in the Framework of Education, Research and Multiprofessional Collaboration – Towards the Health of Individuals and the Society, 7th–8th June 2012; Ljubljana. Jesenice: Visoka šola za zdravstveno nego = College of Nursing; 2012. pp. 276–85.

[42] Gelsema TI, van der Doef M, Maes S, Janssen M, Akerboom S, Verhoeven C. A longitudinal study of job stress in the nursing profession: causes and consequences. Journal of Nursing Management 2006;14(4):289–99.

[43] Tourangeau AE, Cummings G, Cranley LA, Ferron EM, Harvey S. Determinants of hospital nurse intention to remain employed: broadening our understanding. Journal of Advanced Nursing 2010;66(1):22–32.

[44] Van Bogaert P, Clarke S, Wouters K, Franck E, Willems R, Mondelaers M. Impacts of unit-level nurse practice environment, workload and burnout on nurse-reported outcomes in psychiatric hospitals: a multilevel modelling approach. International Journal of Nursing Studies 2013;50(3):357–65.

[45] Zangaro GA, Soeken KL. A meta-analysis of studies of nurses' job satisfaction. Research in Nursing & Health 2007;30(4):445–58.

[46] Lancaster G, Kolakowsky-Hayner S, Kovacich J, Greer-Williams N. Interdisciplinary communication and collaboration among physicians, nurses, and unlicensed assistive personnel. Journal of Nursing Scholarship: An Official Publication of Sigma Theta Tau International Honor Society of Nursing/Sigma Theta Tau 2015;47(3):275–84.

[47] Nørgaard B, Ammentorp J, Kofoed PE, Kyvik KO. Training improves inter-collegial communication. Clinical Teaching 2012;9(3):173–7.

[48] Purpora C, Blegen MA. Job satisfaction and horizontal violence in hospital staff registered nurses: the mediating role of peer relationships. Journal of Clinical Nursing 2015;24(15-16):2886–94.

[49] Moore J, Prentice D. Collaboration among nurse practitioners and registered nurses in outpatient oncology settings in Canada. Journal of Advanced Nursing 2013;69(7):1574–83.

Chapter 7

Transferring Psychological Therapy Education into Practice in the United Kingdom: A Complex Systems Analysis

Ian McGonagle and Christine Jackson

Additional information is available at the end of the chapter

http://dx.doi.org/10.5772/67958

Abstract

This chapter provides an overview of an aspect of a large research study conducted on the subject of learning transfer from an education institution to a mental health service in the English National Health Service (NHS). From a population of 64 trained staff, nurses and other workers, managers and supervisors were interviewed to gain a detailed understanding of how they sought to maintain and develop the new skills and knowledge they had acquired from an education programme delivered from an approved university provider. A total of 45 interviews were conducted using 1:1 or focus group approaches as part of a larger longitudinal study using a mixed methods design. This chapter provides an overview of the qualitative element of the study. Results indicated that whilst aspects of new learning and skill were maintained, many services were subject to pressure to change from the external political, economic and social environment that influenced the delivery of services such as that provided by the one within this study. This complex interaction between the 'external' and 'internal' healthcare environment is an issue that all educators should acknowledge when developing new and innovative education programmes for nurses and other professionals.

Keywords: policy, education, supervision, mental health, complexity

1. Introduction

This chapter provides an examination of the process associated with learning transfer. This process can be conceptualised as the ability to use what has been learned and to maintain this usage over time. To examine this transfer issue, a large scale study was conducted on a population undertaking a new national education programme to instruct health workers in treatments of anxiety and depression using psychological therapy. These cohorts of students from the new national education programme were followed up over a 3-year period to explore the process of transferring new learning in practice.

The World Health Organisation (WHO) in 2013 estimated that mental health problems, particularly depression, will be among the greatest health challenges of this century [1]. Mental ill-health presents difficulties not only to the individual but to their entire social network (family, friends, etc.). Additionally, the economic impact, not only to the individual but also to the wider national economy, is significant [2, 3]. Within the United Kingdom, the total economic costs of mental health are estimated to be £25 billion per annum [4, 5].

Prior to a health policy initiative in this area, it was estimated that only 8% of people with a major depressive illness had seen a consultant psychiatrist and only 3% had seen a clinical psychologist [6]. The unaccounted people suffering with depression and anxiety were deemed to be receiving no form of evidence-based psychological therapy at all [2].

To address the issues above, The Department of Health (DH) proposed by the Department of Health (DH) in 2008 to develop a service to educate and train a workforce to offer evidence-based psychological therapy interventions—the improving access to psychological therapy (IAPT) service. The IAPT service, from 2010 offered treatments, primarily cognitive behaviour therapy (CBT) which increased coping abilities, taught self-help approaches and promoted resilience for future mental health challenges. Referral to specialist services (if needed) could be completed simply, efficiently and effectively. Finally, IAPT sought to promote social inclusion and normal life patterns through access to work. This workforce expansion represented a major investment in education and service development. To achieve this, a national skills-based education programme was initiated [7].

This implementation of a new workforce and national education and training programme merited deeper analysis. It is important that services develop an understanding of the implementation and embedding process for service improvement [8]. To achieve this, an integrative review of the literature was conducted with an emphasis placed on systematic reviews of the 'transfer of training'. Based on this review and detailed analysis of major research reviews such as [9] along with many earlier authors [10–12], key components of transfer were identified such as, the personal characteristics of the trainees, the characteristics of the training programme and the characteristics of the work setting.

To explore this, a series of interviews with practitioners, clinical supervisors, service managers and national policy managers were held. The aim was to obtain a richer and deeper understanding of the process of learning transfer from the national policy to daily practice.

Research on learning transfer models have been primarily linear [10, 13]. This current design articulated a stronger emphasis on a complex systems analysis to understand the transfer process. The study design was a representation of a complex system as it met all relevant criteria:

- A large number of elements are constantly interacting with each other.
- Each part of the system is affected by others, with feedback being a key aspect of its operation.

- Small changes in one part of the system have the potential to create large effects in others.
- The system is difficult to define or boundary.
- The system has a history which helps shape the current behaviour.
- Elements in the system are not fully aware of the behaviour of other parts of the system and only react to what is known locally [14, 15].

2. Method

The method adopted for this part of the study consisted of single hour long interviews with six IAPT therapists who were graduates of the education programme, three service managers (who were responsible for the day to day operation of the service), four national policy managers (who were instrumental in establishing the IAPT service for the Government of the day) and two clinical supervisors (who were responsible for supporting IAPT therapists to maintain and continually develop, their practice skills). Focus groups were held with thirty other IAPT practitioners, who had not attended the programme under review. Focus groups were used to triangulate data from other sources.

The population consisted of 64 post-graduate students studying on the improving access to psychological therapy (IAPT) course delivered at a Higher Education Institution (HEI) approved by the national policy team. The course was a full time, skills based, CBT training course run over a period of a single year. The participants were individuals who had demonstrated sufficient skills and experience of psychological therapy to merit a place on the programme. The HEI which was delivering this IAPT curriculum was approached for permission to seek consent of the student group. On granting of this permission, the students were invited to take part via an email from the course leader prior to commencing the programme. Permission to approach the students was also sought and granted via the university, health service managers and local research and development ethics committees.

2.1. Approaches to analysis: qualitative data analysis

An interview schedule was developed for this qualitative data element of the design. Interviews and focus groups were held with IAPT practitioners, including one focus group of the wider IAPT team from the same organisation (i.e. those IAPT practitioners who were not in the original trainee cohort) and one with IAPT practitioners from a separate English National Health Service (NHS) region in order to triangulate aspects of the data collected. All individual 1:1 interviews were transcribed verbatim and additional notes kept and developed at the earliest opportunity following the discussion. Focus group data were recorded and transcription notes taken from the recordings. The transcription process utilised the work of Kowal and O'Connell [16] and Roulston [17] in taking a pragmatic approach to transcription, with no detailed textual annotations included. This aim of simplicity was carefully considered and so recorded interviews were repeatedly listened to ensure the transcriptions retained not only the documented words but also the spirit of the conversation. Qualitative content analysis used the three stage method for data analysis [18]. This process involved: (i) *data reduction*; (ii) *data display* and (iii) *drawing and verification of conclusions*. All interview data were analysed at a single point with the focus group data integrated a later point to help challenge or confirm initial findings. These processes were achieved by a close reading of the textual material and operating a reflective attention to material even after conclusions had been drawn. It involved a questioning approach to reflect and analyse the nuances in data to verify that conclusions drawn were robust and demonstrable. The emerging themes were developed and refined throughout the process. This process enabled the research data to be interrogated from different perspectives as new ideas were promoted and challenged depending on whether the data existed to support their inclusion. The approach was a dynamic and creative process which enabled other lines of enquiry to be explored [19].

Conceptually, the data analysis approach reflected the examination of patterns in the data, seeking examples with a strong 'fit' with others. The examination of coherence and clustering data aimed to provide a plausible narrative of the data. The narrative could be jarring, but by recognising that dissonant perspectives expressed by participants could also generate important themes worthy of closer examination [20]. The relation between variables expressed as either consensus or dissensus was potential area for the examination of new understanding.

The transcribed and recorded data were read and reviewed many times and annotated. A reflexive approach was adopted to form a picture of the experience of the respondents. As themes emerged from the data, via initial coding and recoding [19] and they were entered into an analysis table and reanalysed until separation of the key themes emerged and the data saturation was evident [21].

In identifying themes, it was necessary to offer a clear articulation of the process of analysis since this supported clarity of approach and facilitates others to replicate the research process. Themes do not emerge within an epistemological vacuum; the researcher played an active role in the process of deciding what is important in the data. Being transparent about the process of thematic identification and promoting a reflexive account of the values and opinions of the researcher, enables other reviewers of the research to assess the completeness of the process.

The research design accentuated the identification of 'patterns' within the transfer process, which are often the tacit but critical elements which play an important role in the complex interaction between organisational structures and process [22].

3. Results

Unexpected findings or extreme results were prioritised for exploration as to whether the study was generating new insights into the transfer of learning. The process of theme development was based on a close reading and re-reading of the transcribed material and a reflexive approach to the research aim. Through this process, a number of themes emerged were considered to have a significant role in the transfer process. All interviews produced a wealth of material and many quotes were gathered which crystallised the emerging themes.

3.1. Theme: confidence and capability in transferring learning

The training programme for IAPT was based on a competency model as influenced by Roth and Pilling [23], although the concept of competency had yet to be adequately defined or measured [24]. Most often it was related to therapist self-reported increase in confidence and their belief in achieving treatment outcomes.

For some interviewees, the training programme and subsequent practice exposure had helped them view their skills more critically. One interviewee, despite having a long history of working as a professional in mental health services identified how the programme had helped them develop a deeper understanding of their skills and deficits. They saw themselves developing new skills and being able to deliver them meaningfully in practice. The process of development was supported through critical evaluation of their skills through the use of video recording of their current competence and capability:

'Just watching myself on video was really uncomfortable, but it taught me a lot about myself and what I needed to improve on'. (IAPT Therapist: individual interview).

The issue of competence and confidence was of paramount interest to clinical supervisors too:

'I think it's probably.....an analogy would be driving.. you can drive when you learn, but you are not used to all circumstances...you should come out of the training knowing what guidelines, processes and treatments are there for people with particular problems. The complexity comes in when people don't fit into those categories, you mightn't know what problem to address and you might not know how to engage somebody' (IAPT supervisor: individual interview).

3.2. Motivation: identity

A relationship existed in the psychological literature between competence, or the desire for competence, and 'motivation' [25]. Within the data an attribute that many responders identified was the need to exhibit motivation to work as a high intensity IAPT therapist.

Respondents considered the importance of developing and maintaining an IAPT identity for the workforce as critical in enabling them to remain within services and remain motivated to develop their practice further. Professional identity and the associated emphasis on personal motivation were critical issues within the transfer process. However, within such a complex clinical environment, significant challenges were identified.

'I have come to see professional identity as hugely powerful'. (IAPT policy lead: individual interview).

'Of course there is tension, our values as therapists are at odds with the managers and the political environment, we know there is the threat to the NHS, so as a therapist you feel quite isolated, there is no shared identity or shared value set, I have no idea what others think because we don't have the opportunity to meet and discuss' (IAPT therapist; individual interview).

Some practitioners identified solutions to the challenges they faced from the internal and external pressures that affected their work. Strongly linked to the concept of motivation and transfer, these practitioners seemed to develop a resistive stance to the accepted norms or a sense of compromise between what they thought they were as therapists and what they were expected to do.

'I work as a Cognitive Behaviour Therapist but I don't do Cognitive Behaviour Therapy with all my patients, I just don't. I can't square that and say that I do. There are some patients on my list, I would say two in every ten, where I do CBT, where it feels structured, where it feels like there is some progression, some therapeutic relationship'. (IAPT therapist: individual interview).

The role of identity as a supportive process to aid a sense of certainty of purpose and to facilitate the coherent and consistent application of key agreed skills and competences was considered important. The national policy leads, made clear statements about, IAPT being an opportunity to develop a new workforce and to protect its emerging identity.

'I think we had in mind from quite early on, they would be part of a new profession. It has developed in such a way that there isn't a professional association for it and that's why it is peculiarly important to maintain the central structure because that's where its identity is coming from' (IAPT policy lead: Individual interview).

The transfer of learning for an (emerging) profession might be predicated on a consistent and coherent application of a body of knowledge. This would seem to be a challenge for the IAPT programme of which national policy leads were well aware.

3.3. Tension and external pressures

The data on identity raised a number of examples where the emerging identity and application/transfer of new skills was threatened by tensions. These challenges were faced by practitioners, policy managers, supervisors and service managers and formed a significant theme in all the analysis. The external wider clinical environment was seen as the principal reason for challenges in transfer behaviour. Clinical practice was viewed as high pressure, time limited and replete with many quotes relating to healthcare provision as challenging.

'Tension is the best way to describe it… between activity, getting people seen and quality, the giving of enough treatment. They have a lot to do… do I think they were trained for this…no! I am not sure you could possibly train people for this… not sure they would accept it' (IAPT supervisor: individual interview).

The external pressures were also evident for policy managers, as the theme of tension was evident in their responses. A number of respondents identified that policy implementation was highly challenging as the 'whole system' worked against an evidence-based application of practice:

'The programme as it was originally conceptualised was about getting CBT into the NHS in more than a half-hearted way, so umm the original concept 'let's just get a load of CBT therapists trained'. (IAPT policy: individual interview).

There were many examples of where respondents identified the shortfall in their initial implementation aims. While on the whole it was clear that many aspects of the policy had been achieved, it had been done so at some cost to compromise and relinquishing control:

'It is impossible to implement something like IAPT in the NHS, because there is always someone in authority who wants to bastardise it, because they don't want to pay for it....there's no respect for research evidence at all' (IAPT manager: individual interview).

The external (political) environment was a feature of every interview. There did appear to be a consensus that while policy formulation was challenging but achievable, the implementation proved a challenge given a lack of infrastructure to support the process:

'Implementation is so hard... these new workforce programmes...because we kind of know what will work but you can't control it, people use their freedom to tweak elements of the programme locally that it becomes almost unrecognisable in the end'. (IAPT policy lead: individual interview).

This was not to say that IAPT practice was not without emotional costs with a number of therapists identifying a sense of exhaustion an often referenced issue within the interview data.

'Well there are two things really. It is a really fantastic job where there are times when I think, I can't do this I'm really crap at it and there are other times when you think, y'know what it's going really well and that person has got a lot out of seeing me.... I am absolutely certain you cannot sustain this, at the end of the week I am absolutely shattered' (IAPT therapist; individual interview).

The time to consider the integration of skills to practice; the process of transfer was not a significant feature of the interview data with policy leads. Yet for other respondents, the focus on targets for client contact and recovery was seen as the main issue about service delivery. It was considered to be the main agenda item at the expense of quality and practitioner development. These targets were the subject of local negotiation and funding arrangements with commissioners. As a consequence, the contact and recovery targets formed an important strand of the tension expressed by managers and IAPT therapists.

3.4. Support and supervision

The provision of supervision was another recurring theme in the focus groups and interviews with IAPT practitioners. Supervision was viewed as a process aimed at providing the supervisee with the opportunity to engage in some form of learning or reflection on practice. In this mode, supervision could be viewed as having the principal role in supporting the transfer process within the work-setting.

Some respondents identified supervision as a management tool used to support service demands rather than individual learning and development:

'the supervision we had during training was really good, but it falls away when you qualify, it is such an opportunity that we don't utilise as it's all managerially led and about numbers rather than anything else' (IAPT therapist: individual interview).

The views of the policy leads varied too on the process of supervision and support:

'I think a model of supervision which is driven by the needs of the therapist rather than the needs of the patient is the wrong way round and we need to stand up and say that'. (IAPT policy lead: individual interview).

In interview and focus group, a number of IAPT therapists stated that originally, clinical supervision was given greater prominence in their working plan, but as workload pressures had increased, supervision had been reduced:

'Supervision is just so…well important I guess. It just feels like we are getting instructions now rather than our development. It can be weeks before you get to see anyone now…not good enough'. (IAPT therapist: focus group).

3.5. Transfer of education to practice in the real world

The transfer of learning acquired or confirmed in educational settings and transferring them to the work setting was at the heart of this study. The 'real world' application had links to the themes of 'tension and external environment' and 'supervision and support'. There was a clear distinction drawn by many practitioners (but to a much lesser extent acknowledged in the interviews with policy leads) between the world of education and the 'real world' of practice. Respondents repeatedly used the phrase 'real world' to describe practice how it *actually is* rather than how it is perceived within the world of academia or the world of policy development:

'I suppose when the university is teaching people certain techniques, they are, quite rightly, saying, these are the rules, this is how to do it. But it is that experience of having to adapt things to the real world'. (IAPT therapist: Individual interview).

This distinction was noted by some policy leads but the dissonance between what was considered good practice and what was evident in the 'real world' was not viewed as a unimportant theory-policy gap. One of the respondents spoke candidly about the challenges for policy leads:

'The distinctive thing about IAPT was that it was highly principled, it was about delivering evidenced based interventions, properly and coherently. It's about having properly trained and competent staff to do that,… and that's what, if you like, makes an IAPT service'. (IAPT policy lead: individual interview).

The issue of transfer from training to the 'real world' or the sphere of influence was an often cited aspect of the interview dialogue. The simple linear development of services and training was not reflected in practice. This simplicity of implementation was viewed as something alien to mental health services, something services had historically failed to develop.

3.6. Therapeutic drift

Therapeutic drift was explicitly and implicitly stated in the majority of interviews. It was conceptualised by IAPT practitioners as the moving away from the set approach that was taught on the programme. The concern was whether therapeutic drift was a relaxation of skills or an example of the development of higher order skills.

All practitioners noted that the transfer of learning had progressed beyond the expectations of training and concern was expressed whether they were still holding a fidelity to their initial training or whether they had drifted away:

'Well…I think there is a balance to be struck, as you grow in confidence, you begin to relax in how you deliver things. I some regards it has freed me up to be less mechanistic in how you deliver things.. the course was delivered in a very strict, almost protocol approach' (IAPT therapist: individual interview).

The reasons for this were varied, but many participants identified the challenges of the external environment as a principal influencing factor.

The issue of drift was also identified by the supervisors, who were clear on the need for supervision to protect the skills that the IAPT therapists had and continued to develop:

'The change, I think in terms of when people first qualify, is that they are probably at their most skilled at that point than they will probably ever be in their careers, er, umm I guess the clinical supervision then..moves to try and keep them, in terms of at that modality level…that focused modality, to try to prevent the sort of drift that is common in therapists'. (IAPT supervisor: individual interview).

4. Discussion and conclusion

The study produced an extensive amount of data which required careful analysis in order to explore the emergent themes. The complex frame used to understand the inter-relationships between the various variables that were used to synthesise the data; to construct a narrative that provided a structured analysis of the evidence on key factors that inhibited or facilitated educational transfer in primary care mental health services.

The results of this study identified a number of inter-connected themes. IAPT therapists, supervisors and managers articulated a picture of psychological therapy in primary care, which was challenging and susceptible to changes in policy direction and practice imperatives. The core target client group; those people with anxiety and/or depression had been integrated into treatment groups with people with additional and sometimes multiple social and health needs.

Data illustrated an emphasis on the desire of all respondents in clinical roles to offer effective psychological treatment and so motivation was a prominent theme. The change model of West and Brown [26] towards behaviour (such as transfer behaviour) identified the need to have the capability or skills to change; the opportunity to change behaviour and the motivation to do so to direct behaviour. According to reference [26], the maintenance of a strong and resilient identity was critical for behaviour (such as transfer behaviour) to be maintained. There was evidence that all elements of the capability, opportunity and motivation process were utilised by IAPT therapists. A number of therapists doubted whether they were faithful to the CBT approach and whether they were provided with as many opportunities to fully practice their skills. The results indicted a link to the concept of therapeutic drift, which again was a sentiment expressed by a number of therapists. Both therapists and supervisors noted concerns that the education programme for IAPT emphasised treatment interventions for anxiety and depression derived from clinical research trials. Many responded with an acknowledgement they were practising a hybrid approach, instilling a sense of uncertainty of either drifting from CBT orthodoxy or developing deeper CBT skills based on the core principles gained from the original training programme. Therapists and supervisors were engaged in a trade-off between practicing with fidelity to the CBT model or developing a deeper sense of confidence and capability in responding to a complex client group. This fidelity drift/confidence dissonance was set within a clearly expressed awareness of the political, social and economic forces at play.

The frequent response from interviewees was that training and its transfer had to be adapted to the 'real world' setting. The education programme within the education institution was viewed as a place to learn and practice core skills in a safe and 'unreal' setting. Exposure to actual practice of IAPT was seen very differently, where concerns of therapist isolation and autonomous decision making were stressors.

The work of Burke and Hutchins [9] was used to guide the research around topics with little or no empirical evidence for their role in the transfer of learning. In this study, clinical supervision emerged as a meta-theme that seemed to unite all others in supporting educational transfer in IAPT. The importance of supervision was mentioned in every interview and it was possible to deduce a role of structured clinical supervision playing an important role in responding to the challenges and opportunities identified in the qualitative and quantitative data.

This study provided an insight into the complexity associated with the process of learning transfer in the English NHS. Healthcare is a dynamic and politicised agenda with many competing demands impinging on the day to day work of nurses and other practitioners. It is important that education developers, teachers and service managers have a deeper appreciation of the complex and challenging practice environment that students are working when considering the transfer of learning.

Author details

Ian McGonagle* and Christine Jackson

Address all correspondence to: imcgonagle@lincoln.ac.uk

School of Health and Social Care, University of Lincoln, Lincoln, UK

References

[1] World Health Organisation (2013) Mental health action plan: 2013–2020. Geneva. WHO.

[2] Layard, R. (2004) *Mental health: Britain's biggest social problem?* London. Cabinet Office Strategy Unit.

[3] Layard, R. and Clark, D. M. (2015) Why more psychological therapy would cost nothing. *Frontiers in Psychology*. Vol. 6, p. 1713. doi: 10.3389/fpsyg2015.01713.

[4] Confederation of British Industry (2011) *Healthy returns? absence and workplace health survey 2011*. London. CBI.

[5] Mental Health Foundation (2010) *Economic burden of mental illness cannot be tacked without research investment*. London. Mental Health Foundation.

[6] Layard, R., Bell, S., Clark, D. M., Knapp, M., Meacher, M., Priebe, S. and Wright, B. (2006) *The depression report: a new deal for depression and anxiety disorders*. London. Centre for Economic Performance/London School of Economics.

[7] Department of Health (2008) *Improving access to psychological therapies: implementation plan: curriculum for high intensity therapies workers*. London. Department of Health.

[8] Greenhalgh, T., Robert, G., Bate, P., Kyriakidou, O., MacFarlane, F. and Peacock, R. (2005) *Diffusion of innovations in health service organisations: a systematic literature review*. Oxford. Blackwell.

[9] Burke, L. A. and Hutchins, H. M. (2007) Training transfer: an integrative literature review. *Human Resources Development Review*. Vol. 6, pp. 263–296.

[10] Kirkpatrick, D. L. (1998) *Evaluating training programmes: the four levels*. California. Berrett-Koehler Publishing.

[11] Kirkpatrick, D. L. and Kirkpatrick, J. D. (2005) *Transferring learning to behaviour: using the four levels to improve performance*. California. Berrett-Koehler Publishing.

[12] Holton, E. F., Bates, R. A. and Ruona, W. E. A. (2000) Development of a generalised learning transfer system inventory. *Human Resource Development Quarterly*. Vol. 11, pp. 333–360.

[13] Klein, H. J., Noe, R. A. and Wang, C. (2006) Motivation to learn and course outcomes: the impact of delivery mode, learning goal orientation and perceived barriers and enablers. *Personnel Psychology*. Vol. 55, pp. 665–672.

[14] Harkema, S. (2003) A complex adaptive perspective on learning within innovation projects. *Learning Organisation*. Vol. 10, pp. 340–346.

[15] Palmberg, K. (2009) Complex adaptive systems as metaphors for organisational management. *Learning Organisation*. Vol. 16, pp. 483–498.

[16] Kowal, S. and O'Connell, D. C. (2014) Transcription as a critical step of data analysis. [in] Flick, U. (ed.) *The Sage handbook of qualitative data analysis*. London. Sage.

[17] Roulston, K. (2014) Analysing interviews. [in] Flick, U. (ed.) *The Sage handbook of qualitative data analysis*. London. Sage.

[18] Miles, M. B., Huberman, M. A. and Saldana, J. (2013) *Qualitative data analysis* (3rd ed.). London. Sage.

[19] Saldaña, J. (2013) *The coding manual for qualitative researchers* (2nd ed.). London. Sage.

[20] Miles, M. B. and Huberman, M. A. (1994) *Qualitative data analysis: an expanded sourcebook*. London. Sage.

[21] Baker, S. E. and Edwards, R. (2012) *How many qualitative interviews is enough? Expert voices and early career reflections on sampling and cases in qualitative research: a discussion paper*. London. National Centre for Research Methods. [Available at: http://eprints.ncrm.ac.uk/2273/][Last accessed 8th October 2016].

[22] Plsek, P. E. (2001) Redesigning health care with insights from the science of complex adaptive systems. [in]: *Crossing the quality chasm: a new health system for the 21st century*. Washington. National Academy Press.

[23] Roth, T. and Pilling, S. (2007) *Competence frameworks for specific therapy modalities, and for their supervision*. Available at: http://www.ucl.ac.uk/pals/research/cehp/research-groups/core/competence-frameworks [last accessed 8th March 2015].

[24] Sharpless, B. A. and Barber, J. P. (2009) A conceptual and empirical review of the meaning, measurement, development and teaching of intervention competence in clinical psychology. *Clinical Psychology Review*. Vol. 29, pp. 47–56.

[25] Deci, E. L. and Ryan, R. M. (eds) (2002) *Handbook of self determination research*. New York. University of Rochester Press.

[26] West, R. and Brown, J. (2013) *Theory of addiction* (2nd ed.). London. Bakewell Publishing/Addiction Press.

Chapter 8

Current Characteristics of the Hungarian Nurses' Workforce

Jozsef Betlehem, Emese Pek, Balint Banfai and Andras Olah

Additional information is available at the end of the chapter

http://dx.doi.org/10.5772/intechopen.68383

Abstract

Recently WHO called attention to the growing labour shortage of healthcare staff, which can reach 12.9 million by 2035. Almost all European countries struggle with a shortage of nurses. The educational structure of nurses has also changed significantly. The aim of this overview is to review the relevant scientific literature and analyse records ofrhe Hungarian nursing registry in order to predict the nursing workforce tendencies. Relevant English and Hungarian international and national scientific literature (PubMed, Science Direct, Hungarian Medical Bibliography) were identified and illustrated with reliable data (2009–2015) from the national healthcare human resource registry and from Central Statistical Office. A qualitative appraisal was undertaken to select the proper articles by our research team. For processing data, descriptive statistics was used. Although migration of healthcare personnel in Hungary is present, however the official statistics does not mirror a dramatic exodus. The level of nursing education is based on vocational training and on higher education in Hungary. The number of novice nurses is diminishing year-by-year and those nurses who are not working in the Hungarian healthcare sector are eminent. Providing new roles for nurses, e.g., Advanced Practice Registered Nurse, can be one of the solutions for the shortage.

Keywords: nurses workforce, turnover, attrition, Hungary

1. Introduction

In numerous countries of the world, including European countries, the negative tendency of human resources in the healthcare sector gives reasons to be concerned about. The WHO

(2006, 2009, 2013) drew attention to the growing labour shortage of healthcare staff which can reach 12.9 million by 2035 and the unbalanced workforce coverage having a negative impact on the functioning of healthcare systems [1, 2]. The Third Global Forum on Human Resources for Health points out that more and more countries meet the minimum criteria of 23 skilled health professionals per 10,000 people globally, but there are still many countries (83) under this threshold. The report of the Forum also highlights that 40% of nurses in developed countries will leave their profession in the next decade due to demanding work, low salaries and few incentives [3].

In addition, the Commission of the European Union drew attention to the needs of nurses in all European Union (EU) countries [4]. In spite of the fact that the number of nurses has grown by 2.5 million between 2000 and 2013 in Organisation for Economic Co-operation and Development (OECD) countries, many countries are realizing nursing shortage [5]. Almost all European countries struggle with a shortage of healthcare professionals, in which nurses are mentioned primarily with increasing numbers in accordance with the report of the Third Global Forum. Across Europe by 2020, a shortage of 600,000 nurses is predicted by the European Commission [6]. The educational structure of healthcare personnel has also changed significantly, both at the level of secondary vocational education and higher education. The conversation between hospital-affiliated nurse training programmes and university level education has taken place in many European countries [7]. Due to the latest higher education reforms, the so-called Bologna Process, nursing education went through changes which can be seen in many European countries. In the European Higher Education Area (EHEA), a full pathway of nursing education including bachelor's degree, master's degree and doctorate title can be evidenced in approximately 60% of the countries, whereas 82% of EHEA countries provide bachelor's degree or equivalent level of education already. However, there are still such countries in Europe who offer diploma level training for nurses only [8].

Based on the OECD database on healthcare workforce capacities in European countries, it seems that Middle European countries have to deal with nursing shortage per thousand population. Only the Czech Republic and Austria report nurses over the EU 28 average. The number of medical doctors per thousand population is over the EU 28 average in Slovenia, among the neighbouring countries. However, these numbers do not mirror the qualitative aspects of the nursing workforce (**Table 1**). The skill mix of the professions, the level of the nursing education, the nursing roles and the staffing are strong determinants of the quality of care. Aiken et al. highlight '*that patients in hospitals in which 60% of nurses had bachelor's degrees and nurses cared for an average of six patients would have almost 30% lower mortality than patients in hospitals in which only 30% of nurses had bachelor's degrees and nurses cared for an average of eight patients*' [9].

The healthcare workforce is a key element of the healthcare delivery system all over the world. To maintain a stable workforce requires more efforts, actions and measures in developed countries. In each developed country, the management of the health sector, the suppliers and the society continuously pay great attention to the development of healthcare human

Countries	Healthcare workforce	
	Practising doctors	Practicing nurses
Austria	6.1	8
Czech Republic	3.7	7.9
Croatia	2.3	5.8
Hungary	3.3	6.4
Romania	2.7	6.2
Serbia	3.1	5.9
Slovak Republic	3.4	5.8
Slovenia	2.8	8.6
EU 28 average	3.5	8.4

Table 1. Practising nurses and doctors per 1000 population in 2014 (or nearest year) (source Ref. [5]).

resources, primarily in nursing. The aim of this overview is to review and analyse the records of the Hungarian nursing registry and the relevant literature in order to present a realistic picture of nursing workforce for the professional experts.

2. Methods: research methods

During the review, relevant English and Hungarian international and national scientific literature (PubMed, Science Direct, Hungarian Medical Bibliography) were identified and illustrated with reliable data (2009–2015) from the national healthcare human resource registry and from the relevant Yearbooks of the Central Statistical Office in Hungary. All articles were identified, screened and a qualitative critical appraisal was undertaken by our research team. Excluded were those papers which dealt with other healthcare professions such as medical doctors, dentist and pharmacists. For processing data, descriptive statistics was used with the assistance of MS Office Software Package.

3. Results

3.1. Demographic structure of Hungarian healthcare workers

In the Hungarian healthcare workforce, less than 100,000 professionals are employed in different posts not including medical doctors, dentists and pharmacists. The majority of this population consist of nursing groups with basic education in nursing and with specialization in nursing. Due to the different terminology used to group healthcare workers, it is very complicated to get an exact number related to nurses employed in the system. Based on the Hungarian Statistical Yearbook in the last available year (2014), 4444 degree nurses (BSc), 14,049 qualified diploma nurses (post-secondary education), 15,205 other specialized nurses, 10,501 general nurses and assistants (now nursing aids) and 1926 nursing aids were recorded in the Hungarian healthcare system. These numbers are controversial to those recorded in the Registry of Hungarian Chamber of Health Care Workers and in the records of the Health Registration and Training Center (an authority affiliated to the Ministry of Human Capacities). The differences of data registered in the different database lay in the method how and what data they collect. In Hungary, all qualified healthcare personnel who obtain a degree or certificate in a healthcare institution are registered in a central system automatically. Those staff who work in the healthcare system have to be registered at the chamber and at the Health Registration and Training Center. At a glance, taking all levels of nursing posts into account, 9.6% of the nursing workforce has BSc degree in nursing in 2014, whereas MSc degree nurses are unfortunately not even mentioned by the Hungarian Statistical Office. If we take out the number of auxiliary nurses from the calculation, the ratio of degree nurses and non-degree nurses is even lower. Sometimes, these figures show a big discrepancy between educated healthcare personnel and those working in the system. After the graduation, the missing persons from the healthcare system have either chosen another profession or left the country mainly, and in some cases, there might be other personal reasons, too (**Figure 1(a)** and **(b)**).

Ageing means a greater demand for the healthcare delivery services. Consequently, the rise in chronic and long-term diseases requires new treatment and organizational forms of caring [10]. Nowadays, the ageing nursing workforce is also a significant phenomenon all over the developed countries of the world. According to the WHO report, around 57 countries struggle with this problem on the developed world. Examining the age distribution of healthcare workers independently from their source in Hungary, all numbers show the same tendency. The changing age profile of the nursing workforce between 2010 and 2013 can be seen in **Figure 2**. The ageing of the healthcare workforce over the age 45 years in the past couple of years is obvious. The healthcare system has to face a salient human resource shortage in the coming 10 years. There is a clear decline in supply of healthcare workers under the age 35 years in recent years. This tendency in healthcare sector endangers the proper function of the healthcare delivery system in Hungary. It seems that the number of people retiring in 5–10 years will outnumber entrants into the healthcare human resource workforce. This figure is even worse among nurses. There are many nurses who work already after retirement; some of them over 80 are still working in health care.

The healthcare workforce is in transition. Clear evidence shows that healthcare workers from Eastern countries tend to seek a job in the labour market of Western countries. Besides medical doctors, more and more nurses think of leaving the country and get a better paid job in abroad in Hungary as well [11]. Those health care workers who would like to apply for a job abroad may need an authentication of medical certificates from the Health Registration and Training Center. The number of applications mirror the intention of health care workers, including nurses as well, who plan to leave the country. Beyond the official number of healthcare professionals applying

http://dx.doi.org/10.5772/intechopen.68383

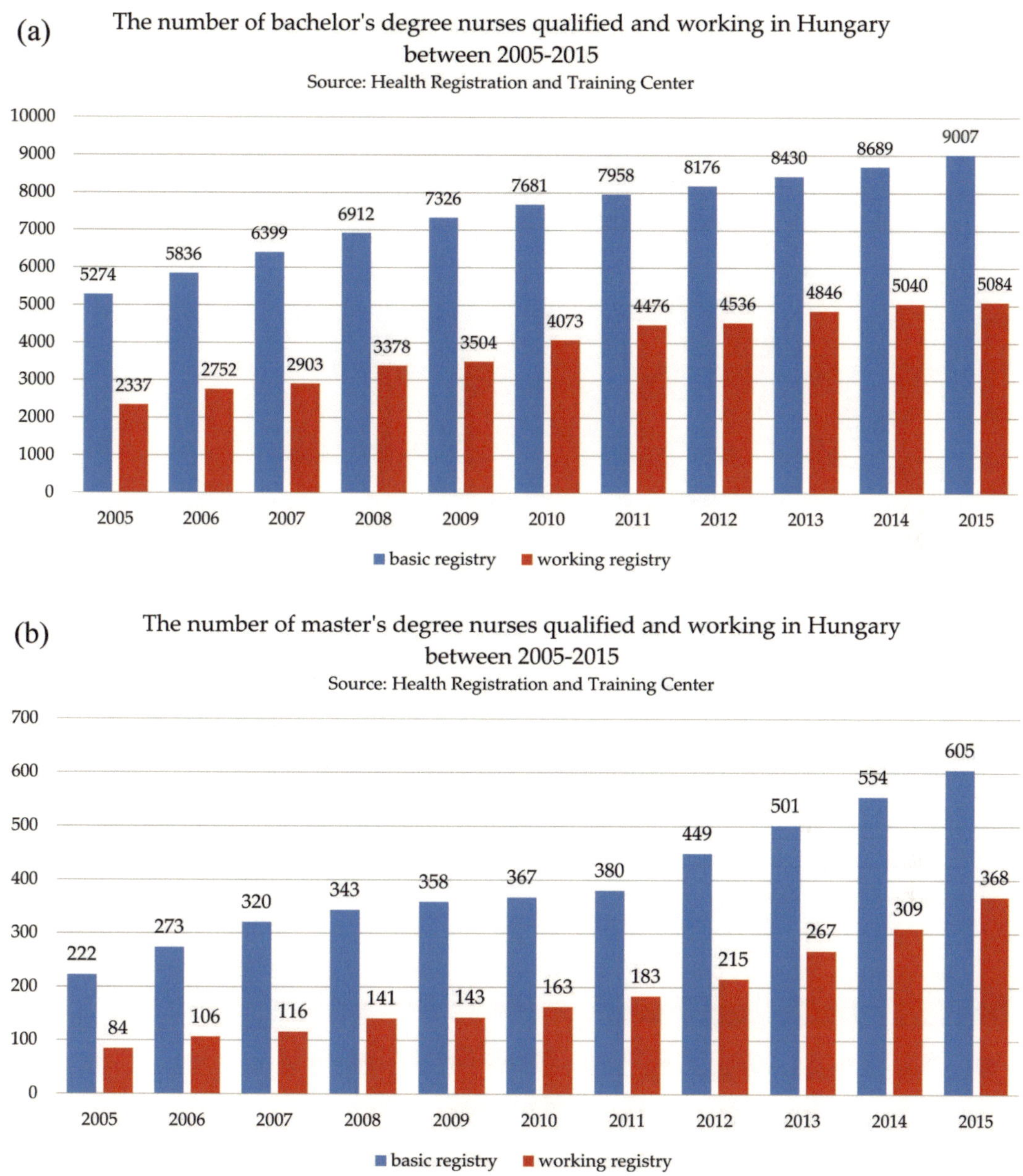

Figure 1. (a) The number of bachelor's degree nurses qualified and working in Hungary between 2005 and 2015. (b) The number of master's degree nurses qualified and working in Hungary between 2005 and 2015.

for a job in abroad at least double as many who are really migrating to west. It seems that we can calculate with a stable number who would leave the country in each year. Nurses' intention to leave the country compared to medical doctors is less, around 500 applicants in each year. In the examined period, the most application among nurses was 526 in 2013 and the less was 301 in 2010 (**Figure 3**). The threats of the human resources shortage and the consequential quality problems

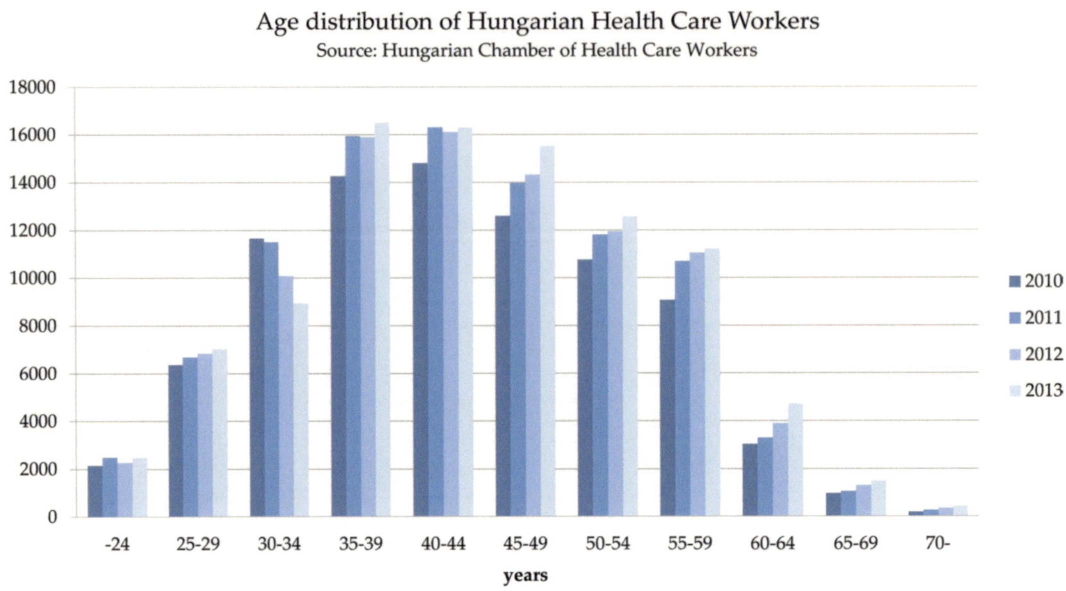

Figure 2. Age distribution of the Hungarian healthcare workforce between 2010 and 2013.

in the delivery of healthcare services are reported related to the Hungarian healthcare system in the past decade [12, 13]. In some other sub-specialities, the problem of healthcare professional shortage is also existing, e.g., in occupational nursing and radiotherapy [14, 15]. In a recent publication, from the Chamber of the Hungarian Health Care Workers, it is estimated that about

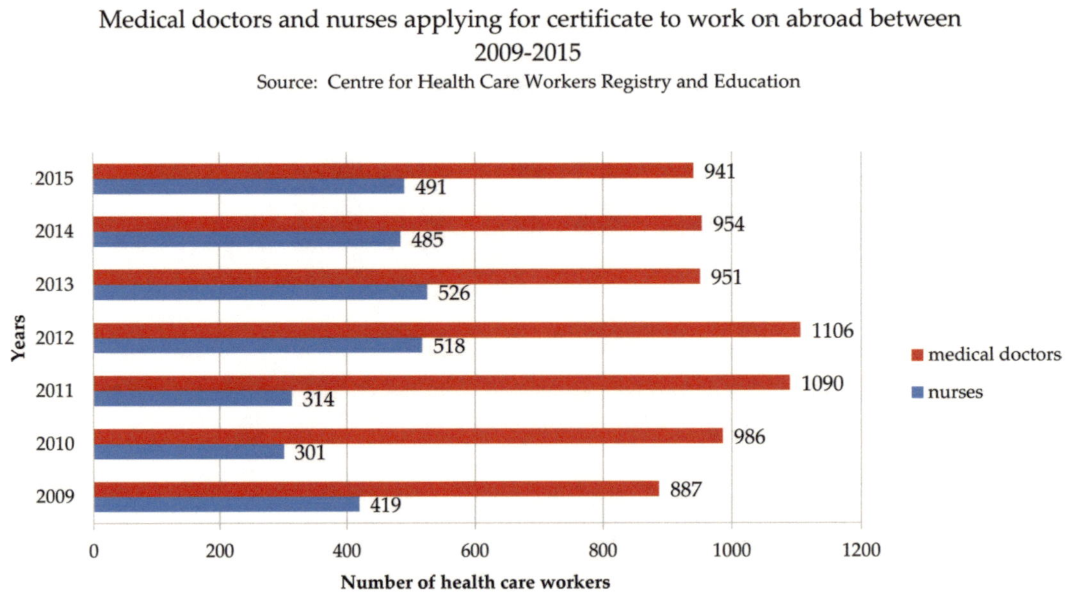

Figure 3. The number of medical doctors and nurses applying for the certificate to work in abroad.

26,000 nurses are missing from the system [16]. Referring to a study conducted a couple of years ago by Ujvarine et al., the Hungarian nurses would need more appreciation from superiors and from society; a better salary and a clear competency would help remain them in the profession. Already novice degree nurses with good foreign language skills would leave the country [17].

3.2. Changes in the system of nursing education

Although other professions in Hungary like dietician, health visiting, public health inspecting and ambulance officer education reached the status of college-level education in the mid 1970s, the elevation of nursing training has been delayed for almost two decades. The transformation of former state socialist countries into capitalism has influenced the educational system, too. The former type of nursing schools initiated by the soviet state still was in function, but new form of education emerged. After the political change in 1989, new level of nursing education in Hungary was established with the help of nursing advisors from United States of America. One of these experts was Professor Doris Modly, the former head of the Frances Payne Bolton School of Nursing at the Case Western Reserve University, Cleveland. With her experience, not just the level of nursing education was elevated to the bachelor degree but also the content was appraised critically and teaching staff further educated. The impact of the North-American nursing education structure showed a 4-year-length characteristics which was implemented during the restructuring of the nursing education in Hungary.

The first pilot programme was started in Budapest at Semmelweis University as a part time education and lasted for 3 years. The later 4-year-length nursing bachelor programmes were launched at the healthcare colleges affiliated to medical universities (University of Debrecen, University of Pecs and University of Szeged) in 1993 [18]. The first master's degree in nursing science was established in Hungary (University of Pecs) in 2000 and followed in Budapest Semmelweis University and later in Nyiregyhaza affiliated to University of Debrecen. This programme lasted three semesters and built on the eight semester bachelor's degree nursing programme. Doctorate programmes (PhD) for nurses have been available from 2006 at those universities where master's programme in nursing is available. When introducing the concept and agreement on Bologna Declaration in Hungary, the Hungarian healthcare higher education was established according to the western structure of education. The conversion from the former educational system has taken place in 2005 as a pilot, and 1 year later, all majors were converted into the Bologna system in Hungary [19] (**Figure 4**). As a later higher education reform, the European Qualification Framework (EQF) was adopted and introduced in Hungary between 2008 and 2015. After the development process, the new learning outcomes were defined and issued by the Ministry of Human Capacities in 2016. The new decree defined nurses' competencies in a more detailed manner according to descriptors of knowledge, skills, attitude and autonomy.

Nowadays in Hungary, more universities are providing nursing higher education beyond those who were starting this type of education two-and-a-half decade ago. The movement from the high-school-based nurse training to university education has also been an essential development of the nursing profession in Hungary, although the newly developed secondary education system takes it at risk.

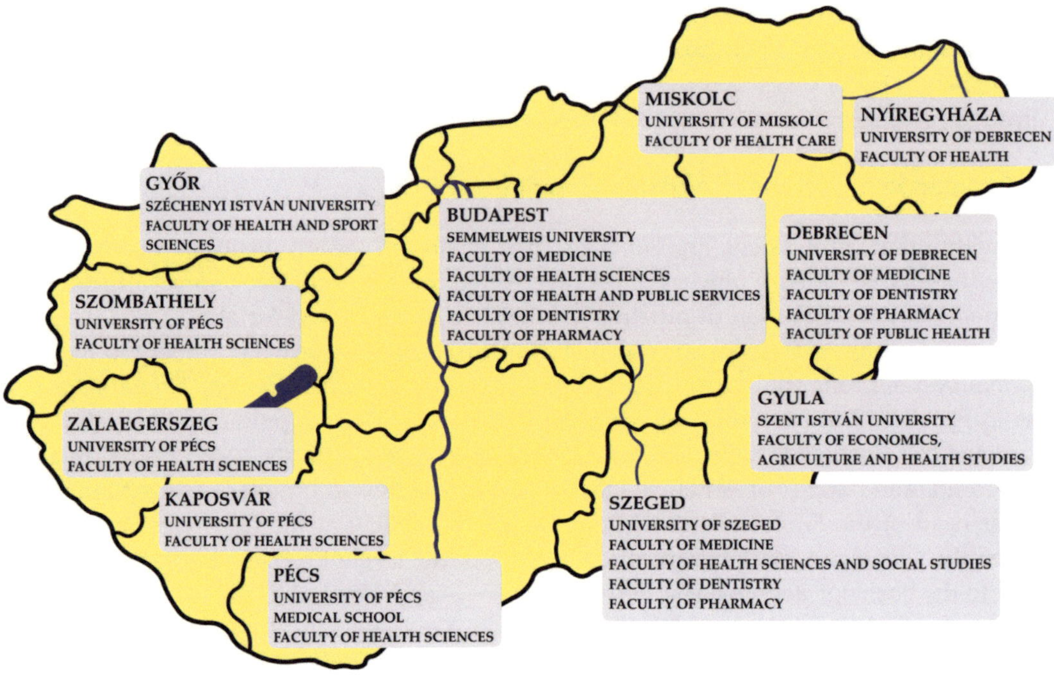

Figure 4. The seats of medical and healthcare higher education in Hungary.

Parallel with the new system, the soviet type healthcare vocational programmes were stopped. This type of education was widespread in almost all of the socialistic countries during the socialistic years. A full nursing qualification was issued either at the age of 17 or 18 leading to general nurse assistant certification. The nursing in the healthcare institutions was based on their work for many decades before the political change in 1989 mainly. After introducing the diploma-level post-secondary nursing education, they were provided with 'birding training courses' to upgrade their qualification. The secondary school nursing education programme introduced in 1997 lasting for 3 years was lifted up to post-secondary (diploma) education requiring a general certificate of secondary education (mature, school leaving examination) [20]. Interestingly, the new Hungarian vocational education reform in 2016 calls back this type of nursing education particularly giving the pupils not just the secondary certificate but a general nursing and assistant aid title. The length of the former post-secondary type of nursing education was diminished from 3 to 2 years.

3.3. The number of nursing students in higher education

Currently, in Hungary, six universities are providing bachelor's degree in nursing (The Tessedik College was merged into the Szent Istvan University in 2008; therefore, they issue the same degree.) (**Figure 5**). In the middle of 90s, three universities (University of Pecs, University of Debrecen and Semmelweis University) graduated a rather high number of new degree nurses, but after 2010, the number of drop out is less than 100 nurses in each year in each institution. If this tendency stays continuously, it will endanger the highly qualified human capacity in the healthcare system.

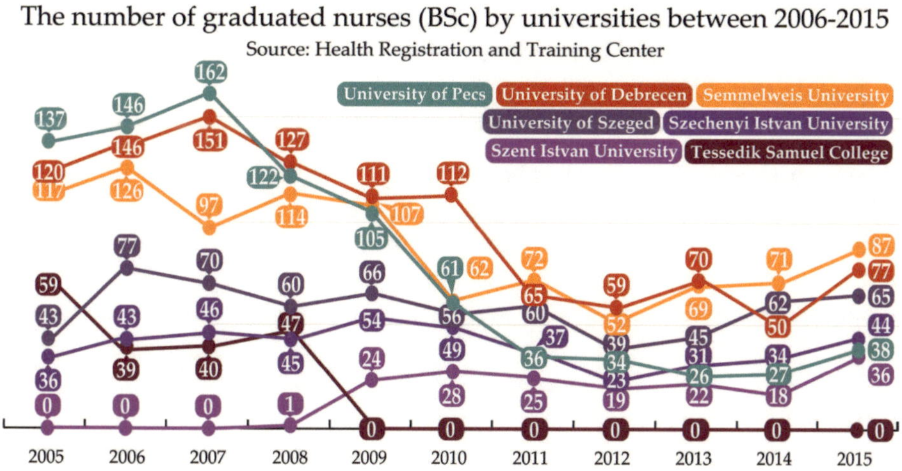

Figure 5. The number of graduated nurses with bachelor's degree by universities between 2005 and 2015.

In Hungary, only three universities provide master's degree in nursing. The number of issuing master's degree nurses is very limited in each year, less than 30 persons in each year. Currently, the proportion of master's degree nurses does not exceed the 10% of nursing workforce internationally, but this number is still very low in Hungary (**Figure 6**).

For young generations who would like to become a nurse, two ways would be available. From 2016, the secondary level of nursing education was renewed. The entry level is at age 14 years. This school ends with a general certificate of secondary education (mature) and a qualification of nursing assistant. A full nursing programme can be completed after further 2 years of post-secondary training. With the age of 20, they can enter into the healthcare workforce. After maturing (obtained in general grammar schools or professional schools), all applicants

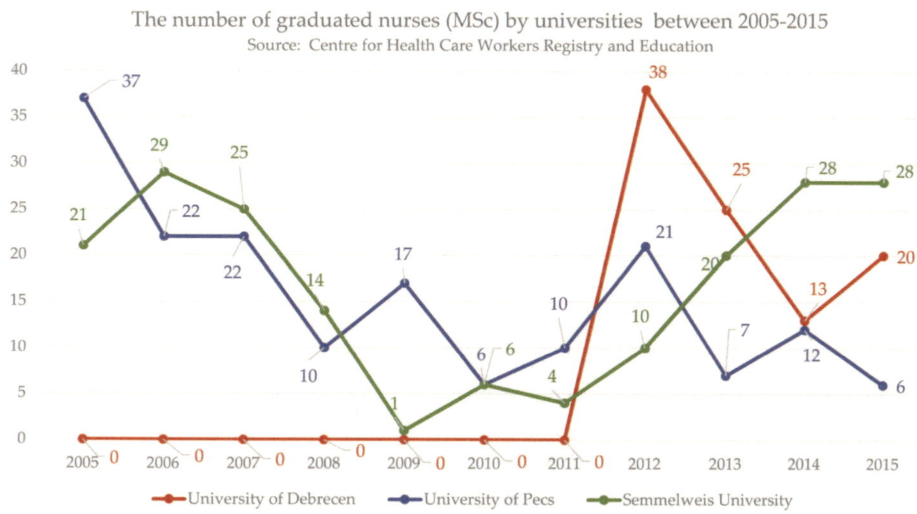

Figure 6. The number of graduated nurses with master's degree by universities between 2005 and 2015.

can also choose a BSc degree programme in the field of nursing. The nursing carrier can be followed with an MSc programme as well. However, these outcomes might be not enough to maintain a stable workforce. From the relevant databases, it turned out that the application for nursing studies is not motivating enough for young people.

In the nursing profession, new role has been introduced in the 1970s. The right skill-mix is a basis for better quality care. The evolution in the healthcare system established an extended role for MSc nurses in many OECD countries. This is a unique role for those who would like to work more independently. This new advanced practice nursing (APN) position is one promising development to help the access to the healthcare system and to a better quality of care [21].

4. Conclusion

In the past decades, the healthcare work force in Hungary faced many challenges. Almost a half of the healthcare workforce includes nurses with different level of qualification. Comparing the standardized number of Hungarian nurses per thousand citizens to other neighbouring countries, it turns out that the standardized number of Hungarian nurses is in the middle range, although it is still under the EU 28 average. In the past 5 years, a diminishing number of posts staffed with qualified nurses/specialized nurses and assistants/special assistants were detectable. Hungary is still among the supplying countries of the European healthcare market. The number of novice nurses is diminishing year-by-year and those nurses who are not working in the Hungarian healthcare sector (i.e., not registered in the working registry and not allowed to work officially) are eminent. Beyond the global tendencies related to the unsatisfied and overloaded healthcare workers, Hungary is also belonging to ageing healthcare work force in Europe. Replacing retiring nurses will not be easy given the global shortage of nurses. Although migration of healthcare personnel in Hungary is present, however, the official statistics does not mirror an exodus. In the past 5 years, around 500 nurses applied for a certificate in order to work abroad. It is still less than for medical doctors taking absolute numbers into account. On the other hand, this out-migration should not be underestimated because other Western-European countries also report about large increase in nurse from Central and Eastern European countries, including Hungary. The main pushing factors are better payment and working conditions. It is also important to retain older nurses due to their experience, knowledge and skills. Sometimes, older nurses have the ability to teach and mentor younger nurses and to withstand and endure change.

Numerous factors have influenced the changes in the roles of nurses and the consequences in the education as well as the impact on healthcare workforce. Since the introduction of nursing education to the tertiary sector, undergraduate and postgraduate nursing education has continued to advance despite changes in the tertiary and secondary education level. In order to impart the levels of knowledge and skills needed to meet the requirements of new qualifications (specializations), new roles and classification for nurses have developed [21]. In Hungary, nursing education remained the 'classical' way of nursing training as a post-secondary type of education lasting for 2 years while big efforts have been made to establish and maintain undergraduate and graduate nursing education. The intake for all type of education is less than the need for new nurses in the healthcare system. In the past decade, a very diverse nursing education system has been introduced especially at the secondary and post-secondary level not even waiting for the 'first results' of the schools. In 3 years, two curriculums have been introduced in 2013 and 2015. Such an intensive change might threaten the quality of training. To make nursing more attractive, pupils should already be informed about healthcare profession at a very early stage of youngsters and a picture about nursing profession should be strengthened in the society as well. Strengthening nursing profession would also mean to show up clear competencies for them and new roles caring for the ageing population.

The new role should imply responsibilities, skills, attitudes and knowledge which should lead to advanced practice nursing (APN). APNs are a quickly growing workforce internationally, growing more rapidly than the medical profession in six countries studied in a research (USA, Canada, Netherlands, Australia, New Zealand and Ireland). Many data on the role of APNs were available in all six countries, however, with variations in quality and role content mainly. Many countries use this role as a potential physician replacement; however, data are still limited in this regard. Growing ANP workforce improves data availability and monitoring as part of the overall health workforce. This information can serve to shape educational capacity, uptake in practice and workforce planning [22]. Evidence shows the APN role does not influence the quality of care, patient safety negatively and patient acceptance, satisfaction proved to be higher. The example of many countries shows that advanced practice roles for nurses increase the attractiveness of nursing as a career, thus providing a solution for nursing shortage rather than worsening the situation. Establishing policy environments and removing barriers will gain in relevance in the future as the demand for high-quality, patient-centred care is increasing [23].

In Hungary, there are many preconditions ready to introduce an adaptation of advanced practice nursing programme and system [24]. The OECD reports that nurse practitioners (a role of APN) programme can improve the quality and accessibility to health care. For an effective implementation of APN in Hungary, there is a need for open-minded health care governing and healthcare professionals. Workforce planning for the future plays an important role for a sustainable healthcare workforce in Hungary.

Author details

Jozsef Betlehem*, Emese Pek, Balint Banfai and Andras Olah

*Address all correspondence to: betlehem@etk.pte.hu

Faculty of Health Sciences, University of Pecs, Pécs, Hungary

References

[1] World Health Organization. The World Health Report 2006 – Working together for Health [Internet]. 2006. Available from: http://www.who.int/whr/2006/en/index.html

[2] World Health Organization. Global Atlas of the Health Workforce [Internet]. 2009. Available from: http://www.who.int/globalatlas/dataQuery/default.asp

[3] Campbell J, Dussault G, Buchan J, Pozo-Martin F, Guerra Arias M, Leone C, Siyam A, Cometto G. A Universal Truth: No Health Without A Workforce. Forum Report, Third Global Forum on Human Resources for Health, Recife, Brazil. Geneva: Global Health Workforce Alliance and World Health Organization; 2013

[4] Commission of the European Communities. Green Paper on the European Workforce for Health [Internet]. 2008. Available from: http://cc.europa.eu/health/ph_systems/docs/workforce_gp_en.pdf

[5] OECD. Health Workforce Policies in OECD Countries: Right Jobs, Right Skills, Right Places. Paris: OECD Publishing; 2016. p. 2.

[6] European Commission. EU Level Collaboration on Forecasting Health Workforce Needs, Workforce Planning and Health Workforce Trends – A Feasibility Study [Internet]. Available from: http://ec.europa.eu/health/workforce/docs/health_workforce_study_ 2012_report_en.pdf [Accessed: 15 August 2015]

[7] Ujváriné AS, Zrínyi M, Tóth H, Zékányné IR, Szögedi I, Betlehem J. The role of faculty and clinical practice in predicting why nurses graduate in Hungary. Nurse Education Today. 2011;**31**(1):94–101

[8] Lahtinen P, Leino-Kilpi H, SalminenL. Nursing education in the European higher education area—Variations in implementation. Nurse Education Today. 2014;**34**(6):1040–1047

[9] Aiken LH, Sloane DM, Bruyneel L, Van den Heede K, Griffiths P, Busse R, Diomidous M, Kinnunen J, Kózka M, Lesaffre E, McHugh MD, Moreno-Casbas MT, Rafferty AM, Schwendimann R, Scott PA, Tishelman C, van Achterberg T, Sermeus W; RN4CAST consortium. Nurse staffing and education and hospital mortality in nine European countries: A retrospective observational study. Lancet. 2014;**383**(9931):1824-1830

[10] World Health Organization. Managing Health Workforce Migration—The Global Code of Practice [Internet]. 2010. Available from: http://www.who.int/hrh/migration/code/practice/en/ [accessed 15 August 2015]

[11] Balázs P. Physicians' workforce and the current impact of international migration in Hungary. Orvosi Hetilap. 2012;**153**(7):250–256 (Hungarian)

[12] Belicza E, Réthelyi J, Kullmann L. Shortage of human resources in the Hungarian health care system: Short-term or long-term problem?. World Hospital and Health Services. 2003;**39**(3):13–18, 42, 44

[13] Szócska G, Romics L. Medical education and the needs of human resources in the Hungarian health care system. Orvosi Hetilap. 2001;**142**(13):659–664

[14] Hirdi HÉ, Hong O. Occupational health nursing in Hungary. Workplace Health & Safety. 2014;**62**(10):421–430

[15] Polgár C, Major T, Király R, Fodor J, Kásler M. Status report of Hungarian radiotherapy based on treatment data, available infrastructure, and human resources. Magyar Onkologia. 2015;**59**(2):85–94

[16] Maleta A, Balogh Z. Report from the 18th Congress of the Hungarian Radiological Assistants. GYEMSZInfo, 2014;**17**(12):8.

[17] Ujvarine AS, Zrinyi M, Toth H, Zekanyne IR, Szogedi I, Betlehem J. Intent to stay in nursing: internal and external migration in Hungary. Journal of Clinical Nursing. 2011;**20(**5-6):882–891

[18] Betlehem J, Kukla A, Deutsch K, Marton-Simora J, Nagy G. The changing face of European healthcare education: the Hungarian experience. Nurse Education Today. 2009;**29**(2):240–245

[19] Kovács LG, Betlehem J. Early experiences with the dual (Bologna-type) university education in medical and health sciences. Health Academy. 2011;**2**(1):57–67

[20] Balogh Z, Betlehem J, Papp K, Tulkán I, Kovácsné Tóth, Á. Nursing education of two decades in Hungarian Higher education. Nővér. 2009;**22**(1):3–12

[21] Ministerial decree of the Ministry of Human Capacities: 18/2016 (VIII.5.) on Requirements of education and learning outcomes in high grade vocational education and in higher education. Budapest.

[22] Maier CB, Barnes H, Aiken LH, Busse R. Descriptive, cross-country analysis of the nurse practitioner workforce in six countries: Size, growth, physician substitution potential. BMJ Open. 2016;**6**(9):e011901

[23] Maier CB, Aiken LH. Expanding clinical roles for nurses to realign the global health workforce with population needs: A commentary. Israel Journal of Health Policy Research. 2016;**5**:21

[24] Oláh A, Máté O, Betlehem J, Fullér N. Introduction of advanced practice nurse (APN) MSc programme in Hungary. Nővér. 2015;**28**:(2):3–10